DENTAL

and

ORAL TISSUES

An introduction for paraprofessionals
in dentistry

DENTAL
and
ORAL TISSUES

An introduction for paraprofessionals
in dentistry

LETTY MOSS-SALENTIJN, D.D.S., Ph.D.

Associate Professor
Division of Orofacial Growth and Development
School of Dental and Oral Surgery,
Columbia University.

MARLENE KLYVERT, R.D.H., M.S., M. Ed.

Associate Professor
Division of Dental Hygiene and Division of
Orofacial Growth and Development, School of
Dental and Oral Surgery, Columbia University.

ILLUSTRATIONS BY MARSHA DOHRMANN

  Philadelphia 1980

Library of Congress Cataloging in Publication Data

Moss-Salentijn, Letty.
  Dental and oral tissues.

  Includes index.
  1. Mouth—Anatomy. 2. Teeth—Anatomy.
3. Histology. 4. Embryology, Human. 5. Dental
auxiliary personnel. I. Klyvert, Marlene, joint
author. II. Title. [DNLM: 1. Mouth—Anatomy
and histology. 2. Mouth—Embryology. 3. Dental
auxiliaries. WU101 M913d]
RK280.M62   1980   611′.92   80-10516
ISBN 0-8121-0701-2

Published in Great Britain by Henry Kimpton Publishers, London

PRINTED IN THE UNITED STATES OF AMERICA

Print number: 3   2   1

Dedication

We wish to dedicate this book to all our teachers, past and present, particularly Dr. C. J. H. van den Broek and the late Dr. E. Applebaum, two great teachers and dear colleagues, who have sparked and kindled our interest in this field.

PREFACE

As a member of a dental health team, the paraprofessional performs certain, more or less clearly defined duties. While it may be evident that groups of future dental paraprofessionals have specific educational needs, in preparation for such duties, their instruction too often does not meet these needs, especially in the basic sciences.

The paraprofessional students are usually confronted with 2 main problems. In the first place, they are required to assimilate large amounts of basic science material in a relatively limited amount of time. In the second place, for many such students, the gap between basic science learning and clinical relevancy may be inadequately bridged.

This text has been written in a manner we believe addresses each of the two problems stated. Each chapter presents basic oral histologic and embryologic information, coupled with a view toward a clinical application in those procedures that the students are trained to perform.

Few students have received instruction in histology prior to the start of their paraprofessional education. We begin, therefore, with an introduction to the *basic* tissues, using as examples the tissues found in the oral region. An understanding of the characteristics of these tissues will aid the students in their study of the somewhat more complicated dental tissues.

Cellular detail, sufficient for an understanding of certain basic tissue characteristics, is presented at the beginning and throughout the text. Since many high school and college curricula already provide introductions to cell biology, the description of cytologic details is a logical continuation of this earlier instruction.

We have attempted to write this text in plain language, intentionally avoiding, wherever possible, the introduction of unnecessary terms, such as the nomenclature of skeletal muscle tissue and the nomenclature of some embryologic stages. We believe that students often tend to lose themselves in memorizing nomenclature, which does not really add to their understanding, and they therefore miss the crucial, much needed information being presented.

We have written this text with the future duties of the paraprofessional student in mind. The greatest emphasis of the text's material is on topics that, from a clinical standpoint, require most detailed knowledge, such as the various properties of the oral mucosa (full mouth impression), surface characteristics of enamel (application of sealants), and the fine structure of the dentogingival attachment (prophylaxis and curettage).

Less attention has been given to other details, however interesting, such as enamel spindles and the various zones of epiphyseal growth plates. Where possible, we emphasize the immediate, practical application of this information.

The intent of this text is to provide students with an introduction to orofacial histology and embryology, which may be supplemented or enhanced by lectures, slide projection and, when possible, laboratory exercises. We hope that this text will provide the paraprofessional students with a morphologic basis for their future work in clinical dentistry.

It is with a great sense of gratitude that we acknowledge the encouragement and capable assistance of the editorial staff and the production staff of Lea & Febiger. We have further been particularly fortunate in securing the artistic assistance of Marsha Dohrmann and the reliable photographic help of Mr. Alfred Lamme.*

We thank our colleagues, who have graciously supplied us with unpublished photographic materials, or have given us permission to use previously published illustrations. Specific acknowledgements are given in the text.

Many colleagues and friends have supported us in our endeavors and have given us day-to-day encouragement. We are particularly indebted to Dr. M. L. Moss, whose assistance in many ways has been essential for the completion of this text.

New York, New York

Letty Moss-Salentijn
Marlene Klyvert

Technical note: The "original magnifications," listed with each of the photographs of microscopic material, represent the ratio between the size of the photographic image on the original negative and the size of the microscopic specimen itself, and should be used only as an approximate indication, since they do not reflect subsequent magnifications and/or reductions in the final reproduction of the photographs.

CONTENTS

BASIC TISSUES; NONDENTAL TISSUES IN THE OROFACIAL REGION

Chapter 1

INTRODUCTION

The oral cavity is a complex environment in which the teeth form but one of the components. It is our intention to introduce to you, in this book, both the nondental and the dental components of the mouth, a study that requires careful observation. It is therefore a good idea to start with an *exercise* in *observation*. This can be done alone, standing in front of a mirror, or in cooperation with a partner. In either case, good lighting is essential.

EXERCISE IN OBSERVATION

With the mouth opened wide, identify and compare what you see with the aid of the diagram (Fig.1–1).

Stick out your *tongue,* move it to the left, to the right and back. Notice how the shape of the tongue alters during these movements. When you move your *lips* from a wide smile to a pout, you will notice how their lengths change.

Now place the tip of your tongue in your *cheeks* and see the bulge on the outside.

With your fingers feel, gently, the *hard palate.* It has a ribbed surface. Going backward your fingers move from the hard palate to the *soft palate.* Remove the fingers immediately when there is an indication of choking. The palate is extremely sensitive.

Stick out your tongue and say "Aaah." If you still have your *tonsils,* you may see them between two folds on either side of the passage way (fauces) between the oral cavity and the pharynx.

Next, take the lower lip between both thumbs and index fingers and gently pull it downward and forward. You now have a good look at the space between the teeth and jaws on one side and the lips and cheeks on the other. This space is called *vestibule.*

The *oral cavity proper* is the space enclosed by the two arches formed by the teeth and jaws.

Gently move the lip up and down and notice that the lips and cheeks themselves are soft and moveable, but that the covering of the jaws is not moveable.

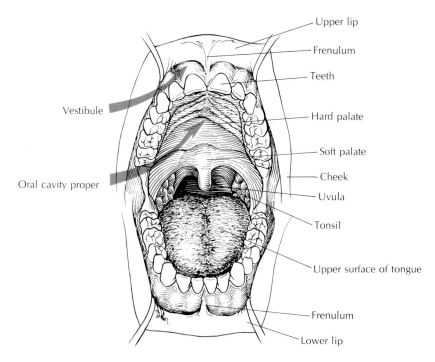

Fig. 1–1. Diagram of a wide open mouth. The two large arrows indicate the vestibule (the space between lips/cheeks and teeth/jaws) and the oral cavity proper (the space enclosed by the two dental arches). Attachment bands (or frenula) run between the lips and the dental arches. A similar frenulum is present between the underside of the tongue and the inside of the lower jaw. It is, however, not visible in this diagram, since it can be seen only when the tongue is lifted.

Repeat this part of the exercise for the upper lip, pulling it gently forward and upward.

Lift up the tongue and place the tip on the hard palate. Inspect the area underneath the tongue. This is the *sublingual area*.

The attachment band between the underside of the tongue and the inside of the lower jaw is called a *frenulum*. Similar frenula are also present between the inside of the lower lip and the lower jaw and the inside of the upper lip and the upper jaw.

Finally, identify and count the *teeth*. A complete *dentition* in an adult has 32 teeth, 16 in each jaw (Fig. 1–2).

Ideally you should find in each jaw 4 *incisors*, 2 *canines*, 4 *premolars* and 6 *molars*. Try to identify, in case of missing teeth, which teeth are missing. Also notice any excess (supernumerary) teeth, if present.

Fig. 1–2. The complete (permanent) dentition of an adult, shown in a human skull. The separate lower jaw is at the left, seen from above, while the rest of the skull, with the upper jaw, is seen from below, at the right. In each jaw there are 4 incisors (I), 2 canines (C), 4 premolars (P), and 6 molars (M).

The "milk" dentition (*primary* or *deciduous* dentition) of a child consists of 20 teeth. These teeth, 4 *incisors*, 2 *canines* and 4 *molars* in each jaw, are eventually lost and replaced by the adult *(secondary* or *permanent)* dentition.

REVIEW OF OBSERVATIONS

In the foregoing exercise you should have noted the following:

Lining

The oral cavity has a pink-red lining, the *oral mucosa*, which covers all surfaces, except the teeth. This lining is kept moist by a watery fluid, *saliva*.

There are many regional differences in the oral mucosa; the texture of the surface of the tongue, for instance, is quite different from that of the sublingual area.

Chapters 2 and 3 will deal extensively with the structure of the oral mucosa.

Hard and Soft Parts

The various parts of the oral cavity have different textures and characteristics. There are hard immoveable structures, such as the teeth, the jaw bones (to which the teeth are attached), and the hard palate. There are also soft, moveable, yielding structures, such as the tongue, lips, cheeks, soft palate and sublingual area.

Even in a small space, like the oral cavity, there are many different components, specialized and adapted for different functional needs.

ORGANIZATION OF THE BODY

The human body's smallest unit of organization is a *cell*. Groups of similarly specialized cells, and their products, form *tissues*. The tissues of the human body, separately or in combination, form *organs*. Groups of organs, related to a specific function, may be combined in *organ systems*. A coordinated series of organ systems is an *organism*. The patient, who will seek your professional services, is an organism.

The oral cavity is the gateway to two major organ systems: the *digestive* and the *respiratory* systems. The oral cavity is involved in many activities, some related to digestion (chewing, tasting, swallowing) and others related to respiration and speech. The organs *inside* the oral cavity are the teeth and the tongue.

TEETH. The shapes of teeth and their hardness are well suited for the breaking up and grinding down of food into particles small enough to be swallowed.

TONGUE. The tongue assists in the chewing process by redistributing the food particles in the oral cavity. It is further involved in the initiation of the swallowing process, and it is essential for speech. On the top surface, the tongue carries a large number of small taste organs, the *taste buds*.

Organs that are not located inside the oral cavity, but are associated with it and important to its functions are the salivary glands and the tonsils.

SALIVARY GLANDS. The salivary glands produce saliva, which is carried via ducts into the oral cavity. Saliva contains enzymes that start the breakdown process of the chewed food particles.

TONSILS. The oral cavity is a major entrance point for foreign matter into the body. Tonsils form a ring of defensive tissue in the passage from the oral cavity to the pharynx.

In the following chapters you will be familiarized with the

appearance of the specialized cells and tissues, which form the organs and organ systems of the oral cavity and its related parts. This study of cells and tissues, usually at the light microscopic or electron microscopic level, is called *histology*.

Part I of this book, Chapters 2 through 7, is devoted to the "basic tissues" of the human body, illustrated with examples of the nondental tissues of the oral cavity. Thus, you will be able to study the histology of the oral mucosa, salivary glands, blood vessels, muscles, nerves and skeletal elements.

In Part II of this book, Chapters 8 through 14, the material from Part I is applied and expanded in the study of the tissues of the tooth itself and the tissues surrounding the tooth, the *periodontium*.

Chapter 2

BASIC TISSUES AND CELLS

BASIC TISSUES

As we noted in Chapter 1, a cell is the smallest unit of organization of a living organism. It is capable of prolonged, independent existence and self-renewal as long as it is in a suitable environment.

At the beginning of human development the future organism consists of one cell. This cell multiplies and different groups of its descendants become specialized for different specific functions. Such cell specialization is called *differentiation*. As the result of differentiation many different tissues develop in the human body, which may be classified into four *basic tissue* types: epithelium, connective tissue, muscle tissue, and nervous tissue. Each of these basic tissue types is further subdivided into several variations. These will be discussed in the appropriate chapters.

Epithelium

Epithelium consists exclusively of cells. These cells form a surface covering. Any surface of the human body that is in contact with the outside world is covered with this tissue type. This includes the lining of the oral cavity, the digestive tract and the respiratory tract, since the contents of these tracts are in *open* connection with the outside world and are thus technically considered as being outside the body.

The further specializations of epithelia depend on their location in the body and their function in that location. An epithelium may protect the underlying tissues against mechanical damage or drying. An epithelium may also be *resorptive* (in the digestive tract) or *secretory* (glandular cells, derived from epithelium).

Connective Tissue

Connective tissue predominantly connects and supports other tissue types. This type of tissue consists of cells and large amounts of

9

intercellular (between cells) *substance,* produced by the cells. The nature of the intercellular substance may vary, according to the nature of the connective tissue.

Connective tissue occurs in a wide spectrum: connective tissue proper, bone, cartilage, bone marrow and lymphoid tissue.

Muscle Tissue

In this tissue type the cells have acquired an extensive and highly specialized *contractile* apparatus *intracellularly* (inside the cells). Muscle tissue consists predominantly of cells.

Various types of muscle tissue, with different contractile properties, are present in the human body: striated, smooth and cardiac muscle.

Nervous Tissue

This tissue type consists predominantly of cells. Most of these cells have specialized in *communication,* the transmission of a message from one cell to the next, sometimes over large distances in the body.

Various types of nerve cells, with different properties, may be found. This tissue is organized in a concentrated form in the *central nervous system* (brain and spinal cord) and in a dispersed form throughout the body in the *peripheral nervous system* (nerves and ganglia).

STRUCTURE OF AN INDIVIDUAL CELL

A cell is capable of performing a variety of functions, necessary both for its own survival and for that of the organism. A *cell membrane* surrounds the *contents* of the cell, which consist of:

1. *Cytoplasm,* a fluid medium, containing many different compounds and small components, such as ribosomes, microfilaments, and microtubules.

2. *Nucleus,* usually the most readily visible structure inside the cell. In this separate compartment, surrounded by its own membrane, the genetic material of the cell is stored. Usually, this material is more acid than the compounds and structures in the cytoplasm, and as a result, the nucleus shows up prominently in stained, histologic sections.

3. *Organelles,* smaller, specialized membranous compartments within the cytoplasm of the cell. They carry out the functions of the cell. Some organelles are the rough endoplasmic reticulum, Golgi complex, mitochondria, and lysosomes (Fig. 2–1).

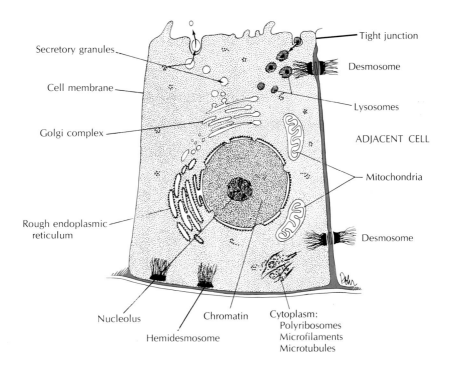

Secretory granules

Cell membrane

Golgi complex

Rough endoplasmic
reticulum

Tight junction

Desmosome

Lysosomes

ADJACENT CELL

Mitochondria

Desmosome

Nucleolus

Chromatin

Cytoplasm:
Polyribosomes
Microfilaments
Microtubules

Hemidesmosome

Fig. 2–1. *The ultrastructural appearance of a "theoretical cell." The cell membrane and the various organelles inside the cytoplasm are indicated. Some of these organelles are involved in synthetic activities (rough endoplasmic reticulum, Golgi complex), some in digestive activities (lysosomes), and others in energy generation (mitochondria). The cell may be attached to neighboring cells by one or several types of cell junctions. Desmosomes and a tight junction are illustrated in this diagram. The cell is attached to a noncellular surface by hemidesmosomes.*

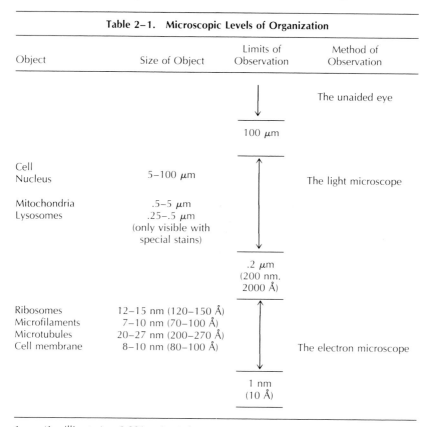

Table 2–1. Microscopic Levels of Organization

Object	Size of Object	Limits of Observation	Method of Observation
		↓	The unaided eye
		100 μm	
Cell Nucleus	5–100 μm	↑	The light microscope
Mitochondria Lysosomes	.5–5 μm .25–.5 μm (only visible with special stains)	↓	
		.2 μm (200 nm. 2000 Å)	
Ribosomes Microfilaments Microtubules Cell membrane	12–15 nm (120–150 Å) 7–10 nm (70–100 Å) 20–27 nm (200–270 Å) 8–10 nm (80–100 Å)	↑ ↓	The electron microscope
		1 nm (10 Å)	

1 mm (1 millimeter) = 0.001 m (meter)
1 μm (1 micrometer) = 0.001 mm
1 nm (1 nanometer) = 0.001 μm
1 Å (1 Ångström unit) = 0.1 nm (somewhat older unit of measurement)

Before we start with a description of the organelles, however, we should clarify at what *level* of *organization* these structures are visible. Table 2–1 should be used as a guideline for the ensuing presentation.

In routinely stained and fixed specimens, studied with the light microscope, the nucleus, nucleolus and a mass of cytoplasm are visible. The other cellular components may be seen only after special fixation and staining techniques and/or with the electron microscope.

Membranes

The contents of a cell (cytoplasm and organelles) are completely surrounded by a *cell membrane*. Membranes are also important

Electron microscopic appearance of cell membrane

Cell
as seen through light microscope

Carbohydrate tail

Lipid molecules
(double layer)

Proteins

Structure of a membrane

Fig. 2–2. The cell membrane is shown in this figure at several levels of magnification. Light microscopically (upper left) the membrane may not be visible as a separate entity. Electron microscopically (upper right) a cell membrane appears as a complex of two darkly staining lines, running parallel with each other, about 3 nm apart. × 100,000. (Courtesy Dr. E. A. Nuñez.) The third illustration represents one of the proposed models for the structure of a cell membrane: a double layer of lipid molecules, facing each other. Inserted in these layers are globular protein masses, some of which have carbohydrate tails, protruding from the outside surface of the membrane.

components of the organelles. These membranes are thin sheets, not commonly visible with the light microscope. They consist of two layers of lipid molecules, into which globular masses of protein may be inserted. On the outer surface of a cell membrane carbohydrate units may be attached to such proteins (Fig. 2–2).

Cell Functions

A summary outline of some of the major functions of a cell and the role played by the organelles in these functions will be given in this section. Please remember that, because of the differentiations that led to the development of different tissues and organs, each

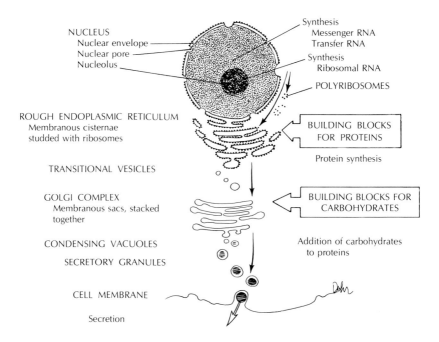

Fig. 2–3. *Diagram, showing the organelles involved in protein synthesis. Messenger RNA molecules, copies of short segments of the genetic code, are synthesized in the nucleus and transported into the cytoplasm. There they form a complex with the ribosomes, produced originally in the nucleolus. The ribosomes appear ultrastructurally as darkly staining, small granules. Groups of them, polyribosomes, are scattered in the cytoplasm. These are responsible for the synthesis of proteins, which will be used inside the cell itself. Other ribosomes are attached to the surfaces of the rough endoplasmic reticulum, where they will be responsible for the synthesis of proteins, which will be released outside the cell.*

  Proteins are assembled into the sacs of the rough endoplasmic reticulum and are transported from there by transitional vesicles to the Golgi complex. Here carbohydrates are assembled and attached to some of the newly synthesized proteins. The product, inside the sacs of the Golgi complex, is then pinched off in small condensing vacuoles and moved in secretory vesicles or granules to the cell membrane. At the cell membrane, the membranes of these vesicles become fused to the cell membrane itself. The product inside the vesicles is then released outside the cell.

group of cells has its own distinct appearance, in which certain organelles are prominent and others may be barely present. There is no such thing as the "ideal cell" (Fig. 2–1), in which all organelles are equally prominent.

Synthetic Activities in a Cell

Figure 2–3 is a diagram of the organelles involved in the synthetic activities of a cell.

NUCLEUS. The nucleus serves as the archives of the cell. The genetic material—deoxyribonucleic acid (DNA)—is stored here in long, coiled strands or chromosomes. The *human* nucleus contains 46 chromosomes. They are only visible during cell divisions when they become tightly coiled. Between divisions the nuclear contents (chromosomes and other materials) are granular and clumped, and they are called *chromatin* (Fig. 2–4,A).

In the nucleus the following materials are produced: *messenger RNA*, which are copies of short segments of DNA, the genetic code; *transfer RNA*, which are molecules capable of transporting specific amino acid units, the building blocks necessary for protein synthesis. Finally, the *nucleolus*, a small distinct component of the nucleus, produces *ribosomal RNA*.

POLYRIBOSOMES AND ROUGH ENDOPLASMIC RE-TICULUM. The various RNA structures leave the nucleus and enter the cytoplasm. Ribosomal RNA is organized into distinct structures, the *ribosomes*, which are visible electron microscopically as dark granules. They may be free in the cytoplasm, or attached to an organelle consisting of membranous sacs or cisternae, the *endoplasmic reticulum* (Fig. 2–4, B). The presence of ribosomes on the outer surfaces of the endoplasmic reticulum membranes give it the name *rough* (granular) endoplasmic reticulum.

Messenger RNA is somewhat similar to a tape that is run through the ribosomes. During this movement the ribosomes act as read-out units of the genetic code. As each segment of the code is read in sequence, transfer RNA molecules, carrying specific *amino acids* (building blocks of proteins) move to the ribosomal surface. Here the amino acids are released by the transfer RNA and become incorporated in the protein that is assembled on the ribosome. Thus, the sequential read-out of the message of messenger RNA leads to the sequential addition of amino acids to the forming protein.

Protein synthesis takes place at the polyribosomes and the rough endoplasmic reticulum. The *polyribosomes*, a group of ribosomes attached to a strand of messenger RNA, synthesize proteins for use by the *cell* itself. They include components of cell membrane and organellar membranes. Directly inside the sacs of the *rough endoplasmic reticulum*, the proteins are assembled by the ribosomes at

Fig. 2–4. A, *An electron micrograph of a section through part of a nucleus (N). Darkly staining clumps of chromatin are arranged largely at the periphery of the nucleus. Notice the continuity of the double membrane around the nucleus with the sectioned, flattened sacs of the rough endoplasmic reticulum (RER). The dark granules attached to these sacs are ribosomes.* × 100,000. *(Courtesy Dr. E. A. Nuñez.)* B, *Electron micrograph of ribosomes, studding the outside surfaces of the rough endoplasmic reticulum (RER). Some polyribosomes (PR) are visible in the adjacent cytoplasm.* × 100,000. *(Courtesy Dr. E. A. Nuñez.)*

Fig. 2–4. (Cont'd)   C, Electron micrograph of a Golgi complex (G). The complex consists of a series of flattened sacs, stacked together, and slightly distended at the edges, where a vesicle can be seen budding off (V) × 120,000. (Courtesy Dr. E. A. Nuñez.)

the surfaces of the membranous sacs. These proteins are for export *outside* the cell.

TRANSITIONAL VESICLES. Transitional vesicles are small membranous sacs, filled with the newly formed proteins. They are pinched off from the rough endoplasmic reticulum and shuttle the proteins to the next organelle, the *Golgi complex.*

GOLGI COMPLEX. The Golgi complex is a stack of membranous sacs. In it the newly formed proteins are concentrated and prepared for export out of the cell (Fig. 2–4, C).

The Golgi complex also synthesizes large carbohydrate molecules and, when necessary, attaches these to the proteins. Finally, this organelle is involved in the production of *lysosomes* (p. 20). From the Golgi complex small membrane-bound vesicles pinch off, forming *secretory granules.*

SECRETORY GRANULES. These granules attach themselves to the inside of the cell membrane, which then opens up and allows the newly formed proteins and/or carbohydrate complexes to be discharged outside the cell.

A

Fig. 2–5. A, Simplified diagram of the structure of a mitochondrion. A smooth outer membrane surrounds an inner membrane, which is thrown into folds. Part of the mitochondrion has been cut away to reveal its internal structure. B, An electron micrograph of a sectioned mitochondrion (M) reveals the outer membrane and the folds of the inner membrane. Between these folds the dark granular contents of the mitochondrion are visible. The contents include enzymes, attached to the surfaces of the inner membrane, DNA and RNA strands. × 80,000. (Courtesy Dr. E. A. Nuñez.)

Energy Generation

MITOCHONDRIA. In order to perform all its functions, a cell needs energy. Cells possess their own mobile powerhouses, the *mitochondria* (Fig. 2–5). These are organelles concerned principally with the generation of energy. A mitochondrion has a smooth outer membrane and an inner membrane, folded in pleats. Between these pleats, and attached to them, are a large number of enzymes, capable of utilizing the final breakdown products of the food we eat and generating energy in the process.

Digestive Activities in a Cell

In order to maintain a tissue, old components constantly have to be removed and replaced by new ones. Similarly, parts of organ-

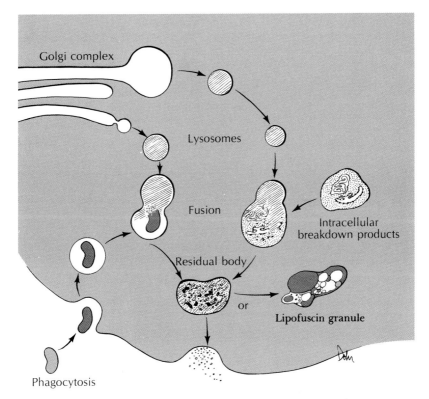

Fig. 2–6. Diagram of the digestive activities of a cell. Lysosomes, containing enzymes, are pinched off from the Golgi complex. Extracellular materials are engulfed by the cell (phagocytosis) and surrounded by a vesicle consisting of a piece of pinched off cell membrane. Intracellular materials, which must be broken down, are surrounded directly by a membrane. Both types of membranous vesicles fuse with lysosomes. The lysosomal enzymes break down the materials inside the fused membranous sac. After the completion of the breakdown process, this membranous sac, now a residual body, may release its contents outside the cell or it may be retained as a lipofuscin granule inside the cell.

elles inside a cell have to be replaced regularly. This is called *turnover.* All cells are involved to some degree in this process (Fig. 2–6).

The organelle responsible for the breakdown of intracellular and/or extracellular "garbage" is the *lysosome.* Lysosomes are membranous sacs, filled with digestive enzymes. Enzymes are proteinaceous substances produced by the endoplasmic reticulum and transported to the Golgi complex. The lysosomes form by pinching off the Golgi complex. If the membrane of a lysosome is disrupted, its powerful contents, when spilled in the cytoplasm, are quite capable of digesting the cell itself.

Breakdown may be extracellular or intracellular. In *extracellular* breakdown (outside the cell), material is engulfed by the cell membrane in a process called *phagocytosis,* and a membranous sac is formed around it. In *intracellular* breakdown (inside the cell), material is surrounded directly by a membrane.

Lysosomes *fuse* with *either* type of membranous sac or *vacuole,* and their enzymes mix with and digest the materials inside these vacuoles. The vacuole with the digested material becomes a *residual body,* which may either discharge the digested materials outside the cell or become a remnant (lipofuscin granule) inside the cell. Many such remnants are found in older cells.

While all cells are capable of *some* digestive activity, some cells become particularly specialized in digestion. Among these are *macrophages* (Chap. 4) and *osteoclasts* (Chap. 5).

Cytoplasmic Matrix Components

In addition to the organelles, other delicate structures are present inside the cytoplasm.

MICROFILAMENTS. Microfilaments are threadlike strands 7 nm and 10 nm thick. The thinner strands, *7 nm* thick, have been identified as *actin* strands. As will be seen in Chapter 6, this protein is present in large amounts in muscle tissue and is involved in the process of *contraction.* In non-muscle cells the presence of small amounts of these microfilaments has been associated with the contractility of the cell, resulting in movements of the cell membrane and actual movements of the cell as a whole, relative to its environment.

The thicker microfilaments, *10 nm* thick, have an as yet unknown composition. They act probably in a *supportive* way inside the cell, somewhat as a "cell skeleton." *Bundles* of these microfilaments form *tonofibrils,* and these converge upon areas where the cell forms attachment plaques, or *desmosomes,* with neighboring cells.

MICROTUBULES. Microtubules are delicate tubes, 20 to 27 nm wide. They are found in cells undergoing *cell division* and also in cells undergoing major *alterations* in *cell shape.* It is believed that microtubules have a *supportive* function. It is also possible that they serve as *tracks* along which particles may be moved.

CELL JUNCTIONS

Since cells in the human body generally are *not* isolated units, but elements of a tissue, junctions between adjacent cells are commonly found. Various types of junctions have been identified. Their structure depends on the function they have to perform.

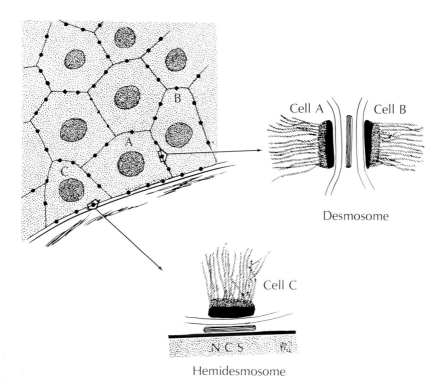

Cell A   Cell B

Desmosome

Cell C

Hemidesmosome

NCS

Fig. 2–7. Desmosomes and hemidesmosomes provide mechanical attachments between neighboring cells and between cells and noncellular surfaces. In this diagram several cells of an epithelium are illustrated. The dots between these cells represent desmosomes. One such desmosome (between cells A and B) is enlarged to show ultrastructural detail. Each cell membrane is represented by 2 dark, parallel lines. In a desmosome these membranes come so close together that their carbohydrate-rich surface coats touch, forming a dense line, midway between the 2 cell membranes. Tonofibrils loop in and out of the condensed cytoplasm, adjacent to the cell membranes. A hemidesmosome is a mechanical attachment plaque between a cell (C) and a noncellular surface (NCS). In such junctions only one cell membrane is present, its carbohydrate-rich coat compressed into a dense line midway in the space between the cell and the noncellular surface. Tonofibrils loop in and out of the condensed cytoplasm adjacent to the cell membrane.

DESMOSOMES. Desmosomes are attachment plaques be-
tween neighboring cells (Fig. 2–7). They provide purely *mechanical*
attachment and might be compared with a pair of suction cups,
stuck together. In these attachments the cell membranes of two
adjacent cells come closer, but not completely together. The
distance between the membranes in these junctions is 15 to 20 nm.
The carbohydrate-rich surface coats of the membranes may touch in

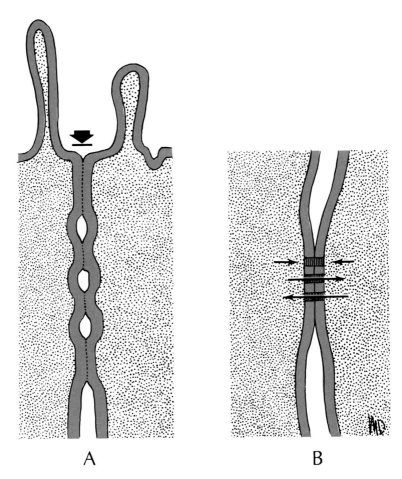

A   B

*Fig. 2–8.   A, Diagram of a tight junction. The cell membranes of 2 adjacent cells (each
illustrated by 2 dark, parallel lines) are fused together in several places. Such a junction runs
all around the circumference of a cell, in belt-like fashion, providing an effective seal. Thus,
it prevents the movement of any substance, in the direction of the arrow, into the intercellular spaces. B, Diagram of a gap junction. In this type of junction, the 2 cell membranes come
very close together, without fusing. Several channels (gaps) through both cell membranes
provide passageways for free transport of small molecules and ion flow in the directions of
the arrows.*

the middle of this space, producing a thin, dense line when viewed in a section with the electron microscope. The cytoplasm near the cell membranes in the areas of desmosomes is somewhat condensed. Bundles of microfilaments, *tonofibrils,* run into these regions. The tonofibrils *do not cross* over from one cell to the next. Desmosomes probably are attachment sites not only *externally,* for adjacent cells, but also *internally* for the supportive microfilaments inside these cells.

HEMIDESMOSOMES. Desmosomes are attachment plaques formed by *two* neighboring cells. Certain cells, facing a *noncellular* surface, may form attachment plaques against such a surface. Since this surface itself *cannot* produce the other half, only one half of a desmosome, or a *hemidesmosome,* results. Compare the structure of such a half-attachment plaque with that of the desmosome (Fig. 2–7).

TIGHT JUNCTIONS. Tight junctions are junctions between adjacent cells, in which the membranes of these cells are actually *fused* together (Fig. 2–8). Such junctions prevent any movement of materials into the areas between the cells. Tight junctions are therefore found in areas where a *seal* is required. In order to be an effective seal, a tight junction is not just a round plaque (desmosome), but a belt going along the entire circumference of a cell. Such junctions are present frequently in transporting epithelia, where the integrity of the epithelial lining is essential, as in the ducts of the salivary glands.

GAP JUNCTIONS. Gap junctions are plaque-shaped junctions where cell membranes of adjacent cells come close together. In such junctions the space between adjacent membranes is 2 nm wide (Fig. 2–8). However, small tubular channels run inside this junction from one cell to the other. Through these channels free transport of small molecules is possible between the cytoplasmic components of the adjacent cells. A low resistance to ion flow (electric coupling) exists as well in these junctions. This allows for communication between the cells and for coordination of their activities. Such communication is essential in certain stages of embryologic development and during activities that require coordination of many cells, such as smooth muscle contractions.

CELL DIVISION (Mitosis)

In an individual organism cell division or *mitosis* is necessary to *increase* the numbers of cells during growth, and to *replace* dying cells during and after growth.

During mitosis a duplication of all cell structures must occur (Fig. 2–9). The most critical duplication is that of the structures in the nucleus. As stated before, the nucleus contains the genetic material, stored in 46 chromosomes. All cells with nuclei have the same

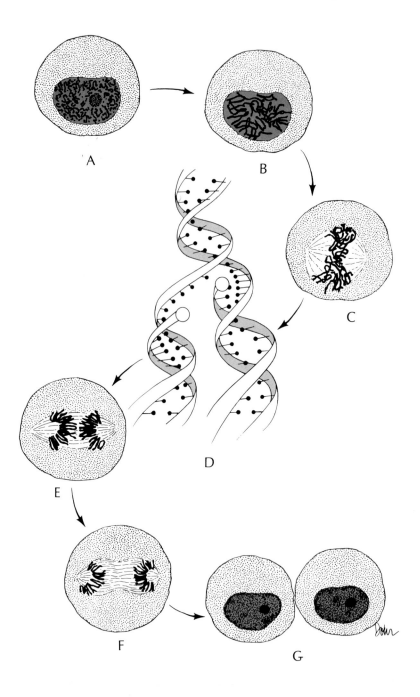

basic information in their chromosomes. An exact duplication of these structures is necessary to give the two resulting daughter cells the identical genetic material at the end of the mitosis.

During mitosis the chromosomes become visible and move toward the equatorial plane of the nucleus. The nuclear envelope disappears. Each chromosome consists of two strands of DNA, twisted around each other. During chromosome duplication, which takes place next, the two strands slowly separate. Each strand builds an exact replica of the second strand. We now have two identical chromosomes. One is pulled toward one nuclear pole, the other is pulled toward the opposite pole. This same process occurs simultaneously in all 46 chromosomes. While the chromosomes are duplicating, in the equatorial plane, a spindle-shaped structure of microtubules is formed. The duplicated chromosomes move apart to the opposite nuclear poles, *along* the microtubules. As the cytoplasm undergoes division, two new nuclear envelopes are formed, each enclosing 46 chromosomes.

The information in this chapter has been adapted as much as possible to the needs of the following chapters. As you study those chapters, continue to review this material, wherever reference is made to it.

←

Fig. 2–9. Diagrammatic illustration of the changes in the appearance of a cell during cell division. A, Between cell divisions no chromosomes are visible in the nucleus of a cell. Some diffuse chromatin and a nucleolus are shown. B, At the beginning of cell division the chromosomes become very tightly coiled and may be seen as strands in the nucleus. C, All chromosomes (dark lines) move to the equatorial plane of the nucleus. A spindle-shaped arrangement of microtubules appears (light lines). The nuclear membrane disappears. D, In the equatorial plane, the 2 strands of DNA, present in each chromosome, become separated. On each separate DNA strand, a duplicate copy of the second strand is formed. In the illustration the growing ends of the duplicate strands are at the 2 points marked with an open circle. All chromosomes are duplicated in this way. E, One of each of all duplicated sets of chromosomes is now pulled along the microtubular frame in opposite directions. F, In this stage 46 chromosomes are present at each of the 2 opposite poles of the microtubular spindle. G, The spindle disappears. Both groups of chromosomes are surrounded by a nuclear membrane. Once the 2 nuclei are thus formed, the cytoplasm undergoes division and 2 "daughter cells" are formed, essentially similar to the original "mother cell."

SELECTED READING LIST

The Cell and Its Functions

Bloom, W., and Fawcett, D. W.: The cell and cell division. In *A Textbook of Histology*. 10th Ed. Philadelphia, W. B. Saunders Co., 1975.

Bourne, G. H.: *Division of Labor in Cells*. 2nd Ed. New York, Academic Press, 1970.

Fawcett, D. W.: *An Atlas of Fine Structure. The Cell, Its Organelles and Inclusions*. Philadelphia, W. B. Saunders Co., 1966.

Holtzman, E., and Novikoff, A. B.: *Cells and Organelles*. New York, Holt, Rinehart and Winston, Inc., 1970.

Hopkins, C.R.: *Structure and Function of Cells*. Philadelphia, W.B. Saunders Co., 1978.

Lentz, T.: *Cell Fine Structure. An Atlas of Drawings of Whole Cell Structure*. Philadelphia, W.B. Saunders Co., 1971.

Mazia, D.: The cell cycle. Sci. Am., *230*:54, 1974.

Porter, K.R., and Bonneville, M.A.: *Fine Structure of Cells and Tissues*. Philadelphia, Lea & Febiger, 1968.

Cell Membranes

Bretscher, M.S.: Membrane structure: some general principles. Science, *181*:622, 1973.

Capaldi, R.A.: A dynamic model of cell membranes. Sci. Am., *230*:26, 1974.

Parsons, D.F., and Subjeck, J.R.: Morphology of the polysaccharide coat of mammalian cells. Biochim. Biophys. Acta, *265*:85, 1972.

Singer, S.J., and Nicolson, G.L.: The fluid mosaic model of the structure of cell membranes. Science, *175*:720, 1972.

Cell Junctions

Bloom, W., and Fawcett, D.W.: Epithelium. In *A Textbook of Histology*. 10th Ed. Philadelphia, W.B. Saunders Co., 1975.

Goodenough, D.A., and Revel, J.P.: A fine structural analysis of intercellular junctions in the mouse liver. J. Cell Biol., *45*:272, 1970.

Peracchia, C.: Gap junction structure and function. Trends in Biochemical Sciences, Feb. 1977.

Chapter 3

THE ORAL MUCOSA—EPITHELIUM

In Chapter 1 we found that there are variations in appearance, structure and texture of the various parts of the oral cavity. We shall now study more precisely the appearance of the *lining* of the oral cavity, the *oral mucosa*.

Inspect, once more, the area of the oral vestibule by gently pulling the lower lip downward and forward. Compare your observations with the structures indicated in Figure 3–1. Using these figures as a guide, locate the following in your own mouth: *interdental papillae,* bulges of oral mucosa between adjacent teeth; *free gingiva,* the strip of about 1.5 mm along the edge of gingiva; *free gingival line,* borderline between free and attached gingivae; *attached gingiva,* the gingiva directly overlying the bone of the jaw; *mucogingival line,* borderline between attached gingiva and alveolar mucosa; *alveolar mucosa,* the mucosa covering the floor of the vestibule; and *labial mucosa,* the mucosa covering the inside of the lip.

Compare the color and texture of the *attached gingiva* with those of the *alveolar* and *labial mucosae.* Which is redder? Which looks moister? Notice the relatively sharp lines between free and attached gingivae (the *free gingival line*) and between attached gingiva and alveolar mucosa (the *mucogingival line*).

Now, move the lip gently up and down and see to what extent the mucosa may be moved.

Ideally, you should have noted that the *attached gingiva* is generally lighter and pinker in color than the *alveolar* and *labial mucosae.* If the gingiva is healthy, it may have a slightly pitted, "orange peel" appearance. The alveolar and labial mucosae look somewhat moister than the gingiva. When the lip is pulled, the alveolar and labial mucosae are moved along, but the motion stops at the mucogingival line.

The attached gingiva is strongly tied to the underlying tissue—the bone of the jaw. It is difficult to compress the attached gingiva and it cannot be shifted from left to right or up and down, relative to the underlying bony structures. On the other hand, the labial mucosa

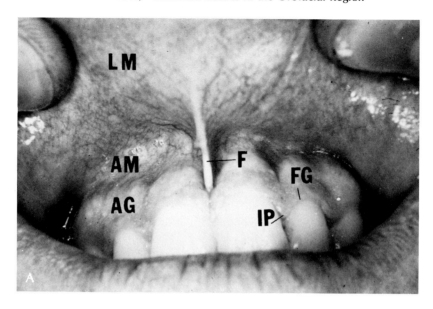

Fig. 3–1.   Part of the oral vestibule is shown in this photograph. The upper front teeth and a frenulum (F) are prominently visible. IP = interdental papilla; FG = free gingiva; AG = attached gingiva; AM = alveolar mucosa; LM = labial mucosa. (Courtesy Dr. E.V. Zegarelli.)

may be compressed readily. When released it jumps back. The labial mucosa may be easily shifted back and forth over the underlying tissues, that is, muscles and salivary glands.

You have just seen good examples of two types of oral mucosa—the attached gingiva is an example of *masticatory* mucosa; labial and alveolar mucosae are examples of *lining* mucosa.

Actually, we distinguish *three* types of mucosae in the oral cavity (Fig. 3–2): (1) *lining mucosa*, the lining of cheeks and lips (*buccal* and *labial* mucosae), soft palate and sublingual area; (2) *masticatory mucosa*, the lining of attached gingiva and of hard palate; and (3) *specialized mucosa*, the lining of the top surface of the tongue, which carries specialized papillae, some with *taste buds*.

Clinically, the distinction between lining and masticatory mucosae is important. Let us illustrate this with the following exercise.

Place your fingers in the oral vestibule, between upper jaw and upper lip. Now, with the finger in place, vigorously move the lip in

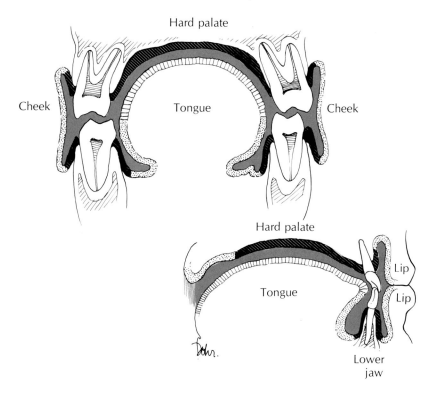

Fig. 3–2. *Two diagrams showing the distribution of the three types of mucosa in the oral cavity. The top figure represents a section from side to side through the tissues of the mouth, while the bottom figure illustrates a midline section from back to front. The stippled areas are covered with lining mucosa. The darkly hatched areas are covered with masticatory mucosa. The top of the tongue is covered with specialized mucosa.*

all directions. You will notice that the only stable region is that of the attached gingiva. Repeat this exercise by placing your finger against the inner surface of the lower jaw, behind the incisors. With the finger in place, move the tongue in all directions. Again, you will find that the only stable region is that of the attached gingiva. Select as many areas of the oral cavity as possible, to repeat this exercise. You will find that only the *attached gingivae* and the *lining* of the *hard palate,* the areas covered with *masticatory mucosa,* are stable.

A full denture, or any other prosthetic device, which rests on an area of oral mucosa, needs a stable surface for optimal functioning. A successful denture therefore, should not only fit well, it should also be supported exclusively by masticatory mucosa. If it does extend further, onto areas of lining mucosa, it will become unseated during the movements of the soft tissues. This distinction is so important that in the first impression taken for the construction of a prosthesis, the lines separating lining and masticatory mucosae are indicated as a guide for subsequent procedures.

STRUCTURE OF THE ORAL MUCOSA

The oral mucosa consists of *two basic tissues*—the *epithelium* or superficial layer and *connective tissue* or the underlying, supporting layer.

A cut through the thickness of the oral mucosa shows features that are in many ways similar to those of the skin (Fig. 3–3):

1. The superficial layer of the oral mucosa is the *oral epithelium;* the superficial layer of the skin is the *epidermis* (epithelium).

2. The supporting connective tissue layer in the oral mucosa is the *lamina propria;* a similar layer in the skin is the *dermis.*

3. Underneath the oral mucosa in some areas a *submucosa* (connective tissue) is found; a similar connective tissue structure is usually present underneath the skin: the *hypodermis.*

While the skin has some particular specializations, such as hairs, nails and sweat glands, which are not found in the oral mucosa, the type of epithelium, as well as the nature and the arrangement of the connective tissue layers, are similar in skin and oral mucosa.

The oral epithelium forms a mechanical barrier protecting the underlying tissues. The connective tissue forms a mechanical support, because of its structural density and arrangement, but it also carries the vital supply systems to the region—the blood vessels and the nerves.

While a more complete listing of the *regional differences* between lining, masticatory and specialized mucosae may be found at the end of Chapter 4, we should note here the *principal* characteristics of each of these oral mucosa types (Fig. 3–4).

LINING MUCOSA. The epithelial layer of this type of mucosa usually consists of nonkeratinized, stratified squamous epithelium (this chapter). The interface between epithelium and connective tissue is gently undulated. Relatively few short and broad connective tissue extensions *(papillae)* project into the epithelial layer. A lining mucosa is generally compressible and moveable, relative to the underlying tissue, a characteristic that is due to the presence of a submucosa between lamina propria and that underlying tissue (usually muscle tissue).

MASTICATORY MUCOSA. The epithelial layer of this type of mucosa usually consists of keratinized stratified squamous epithelium. The interface between epithelium and connective tissue is strongly interdigitated: many tall, narrow connective tissue papillae project into the epithelium. Alternating with these are usually as many tall, thin epithelial extensions *(rete pegs)*, projecting

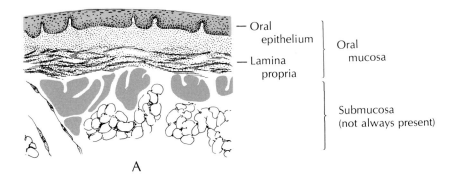

— Oral
  epithelium
— Lamina
  propria

Oral
mucosa

Submucosa
(not always present)

A

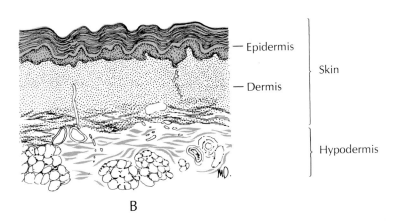

— Epidermis

— Dermis

Skin

Hypodermis

B

Fig. 3–3. In these 2 diagrams a comparison is made between the appearances of sections through oral mucosa (A) and skin (B). The oral epithelium and the epidermis are the superficial epithelial layers. The lamina propria and the dermis are the highly organized connective tissue layers underneath the epithelium layers. The submucosa (not always present) and the hypodermis are somewhat more loosely organized connective tissue layers, located between oral mucosa or skin and the underlying tissues (muscles, bones).

LINING MUCOSA   MASTICATORY MUCOSA   SPECIALIZED MUCOSA

Muscle

Bone

Tongue muscles

Fig. 3–4. Diagram of the general characteristics of the 3 types of oral mucosae. Highlighted are the differences in epithelial thickness, degree of epithelial keratinization, thickness of lamina propria, shapes of connective tissue papillae and presence or absence of a submucosa.

into the underlying connective tissue. A submucosa is usually absent. The lamina propria is tied strongly and directly to the underlying tissue (generally bone). A masticatory mucosa is largely resistant to compression and immoveable, relative to the underlying tissue. This is a mechanically strong lining, capable of withstanding masticatory loading.

SPECIALIZED MUCOSA. This type of mucosa is found on the top surface of the tongue *only,* and it forms distinct specializations, *lingual papillae,* some of which carry *taste buds.* The stratified squamous epithelium of the tongue varies in thickness and in degree of keratinization. The connective tissue forms the extensive and specialized lingual papillae. There is no submucosa; the specialized mucosa is tied directly to the underlying muscles of the tongue. This makes the specialized mucosa immoveable relative to these muscles and allows it to conform precisely to the movements of these muscles. The three different types of oral mucosa are illustrated schematically in their most general form in Figure 3–4.

EPITHELIUM

Despite the existence of many different types of epithelium, all types have in common the following characteristic: epithelium consists of a layer of cells in close contact with each other over a large part of their cell surfaces, with little intercellular space.

Epithelia may be *classified* according to their *function* as (1) a protective barrier (examples: epidermis, oral epithelium), (2) a group of secretory cells (example: epithelium of salivary glands), (3) a group of resorbing cells (example: gut epithelium), and (4) a group of cells of special sense (example: taste cells).

Another commonly used and simple way to describe the various types of epithelia is by using two morphologic characteristics:

1. The *shapes* of the *most superficial* cells of an epithelium. We distinguish three shapes (Fig. 3–5)—flat *(squamous)*, cuboidal, and columnar.

2. The *number of cell layers* in an epithelium. An epithelium may consist of *one* cell layer (a *simple* epithelium) or of *several* cell layers (a *stratified* epithelium).

Using combinations of these distinguishing morphologic characteristics, six different types of epithelium may be described: simple squamous, simple cuboidal, simple columnar, stratified squamous, stratified cuboidal and stratified columnar. Add to these combinations some intermediate forms, as well as some surface specializations, and you will have some appreciation of the variations in epithelial tissues. The various differences in epithelial cells are related to their different functions in different locations of the body.

ORAL EPITHELIUM

Oral epithelium in the oral mucosa and epidermis in the skin are examples of *stratified squamous epithelia.*

The main functions of such epithelia are *protective.* They form protective barriers against mechanical insults, bacterial invasions and, in the epidermis, loss of tissue fluids.

Stratified squamous epithelia consist of constantly renewing cell populations. Under normal conditions the rate of cell loss from the superficial layers of the epithelia matches the rate of new cell production by mitosis in the deepest layers of these epithelia. During the aging process each cell moves slowly up from the deepest *(basal)* layer to the more superficial layers, where it finally becomes detached. Thus, in a certain time span, an epithelium may be entirely replaced by a new cell generation. This time span, or *turnover time,* has been studied for some regions of the human epidermis and oral epithelium. Turnover times in the epidermis range from 12 to 75 days. Turnover times for the oral epithelium of

Squamous

Cuboidal

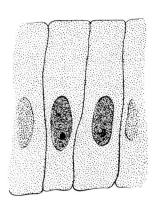

Columnar

Fig. 3–5.   Principal morphologic characteristics of epithelial cells: squamous cells (flat), cuboidal cells and columnar cells. While the cuboidal and columnar cells are shown here in one cell layer (simple epithelium), the squamous cells are illustrated in an arrangement of several cell layers, stacked together (stratified epithelium).

the cheek (buccal epithelium) range from 5 to 16 days. The turnover times for the epithelium of the hard palate and the sublingual region are slightly longer, but still shorter than for the epidermis.

Since the superficial cells of the oral epithelium are readily detached, it is relatively simple to remove some of them from your own mouth and study them with the light microscope (see Appendix 1 for instructions on the use of the microscope).

Move the tip of your tongue or a cotton swab over the inside of your cheek. Then touch the center of a glass slide *lightly* with tongue tip or cotton swab. Place an even smaller and thinner glass cover *(cover glass)* over the area of the glass slide you just touched. The preparation is now ready for study under the microscope. For better visibility of the structures you want to study under the microscope, the area with the material from the oral cavity may be stained with a histologic dye, such as methylene blue.

Under the microscope, your preparation will show several small, flattened structures. These are the detached superficial cells from the oral epithelium. These cells are predominantly flat and

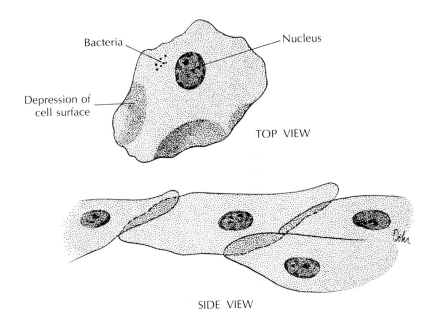

Fig. 3–6. Diagram of the appearance of a nonkeratinized, squamous epithelial cell, following its removal from the oral cavity and the histologic preparation, described in the text. In the flat, pancake-shaped cell a nucleus is usually visible and occasionally some bacteria on the cell surface. Where the cell was compressed against neighboring epithelial cells, depressions of the cell surface are present. The bottom diagram illustrates how several epithelial cells may be pressed together to create such depressions on their surfaces.

pancake-shaped and have given the epithelium its classification: *squamous*. The cells clearly show how closely they have been compressed against their neighboring cells prior to being moved to your glass slide. They actually have little depressions on their surfaces. If the cells are properly stained, you may see an ovoid to rounded nucleus, roughly in the center of the cells, and variable numbers of bacteria, visible as tiny, darkly stained dots, on the cell surfaces. The latter are members of the normal bacterial population of the mouth (Fig. 3–6).

Depending on their location, stratified squamous epithelia may or may not become cornified *(keratinized)* in their superficial layers. We distinguish three forms of stratified squamous epithelia.

1. (Ortho)*keratinized* stratified squamous epithelium. This is found in the skin and in some parts of the masticatory and specialized mucosae. The keratinization is effective for mechanical protection, but it acts especially to produce a barrier against fluid loss. If present in the oral cavity, this type of stratified squamous epithelium is the *least* frequently found of these three.

2. *Nonkeratinized* stratified squamous epithelium. This is found in the mouth, in the areas of the lining mucosa. It acts as a cushion, protecting against mechanical damage, and as a selective barrier.

3. *Parakeratinized* stratified squamous epithelium. This is a middle form between orthokeratinized and nonkeratinized epithelia. It is found in the mouth: in most of the masticatory mucosa and in some of the specialized mucosa.

Layers in Stratified Squamous Epithelia

As stated previously, cell divisions occur in the basal layer of the stratified squamous epithelia, while cells of the superficial layer become detached and are lost. In its journey from the basal layer to the most superficial layer, an epithelial cell undergoes definite *maturational* changes, and since all its neighbors in the same horizontal plane undergo the same changes, there are morphologically distinct zones or *layers* in a stratified squamous epithelium. These layers, in order, are (Fig. 3–7):

BASAL LAYER (deepest). The cells in it are cuboidal in shape and they regularly undergo cell divisions. This layer consists of one single cell layer.

PRICKLE CELL LAYER. This name is given because the cells in it, which are polygonal in shape, have a "spiky" appearance. This appearance is the result of the histologic fixation, which frequently causes shrinkage of the cells.

A cell may shrink in all areas where it does *not* form a junction with neighboring cells. The locations where junctions *(desmosomes)* are present are prevented from pulling away as a result of the shrinkage. They form the spikes. The prickle cell layer is several cell layers thick.

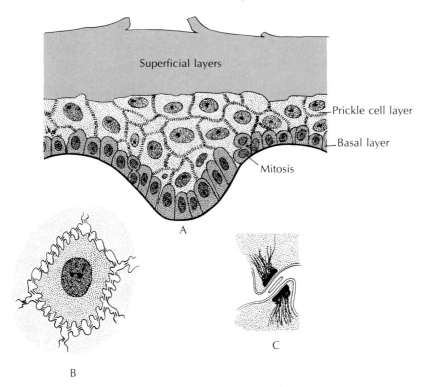

Superficial layers

Prickle cell layer

Basal layer

Mitosis

A

B

C

Fig. 3–7. A, *Histologic appearance of the deeper layers of the 3 types of stratified squamous epithelia. Thicknesses of such layers may vary locally, but generally both are present. The superficial layers, which are different in the 3 types of epithelia, have been left blank in this diagram. The basal layer is the deepest layer, adjacent to the connective tissue. These cells stain darkly and undergo continued mitoses. Some mitoses are indicated here. The prickle cell layer, above the basal layer, consists of polygonal cells. B, A single cell of the prickle cell layer is shown. The spikes on the cell surface make contact with similar spikes on the neighboring cell surfaces. These contacts consist of desmosomes, one of which is illustrated in C. The desmosomes themselves are not visible with the light microscope, but the spikes, produced by fixation shrinkage, indicate the desmosome locations.*

In the three different types of stratified squamous epithelia, the two layers just described are always present. They account for about one half to two thirds of the total epithelial thickness, and they have approximately the same appearance in these three types. All three epithelia, furthermore, have a well-developed *internal,* intracellular support system of *tonofibrils,* suitable for their mechanical functions. These tonofibrils are well-organized *bundles* of 10 nm thick microfilaments, running inside the cytoplasm of the epithelial cells and attaching into the areas of the desmosomes.

In their more *superficial* layers, the three forms of stratified squamous epithelia exhibit a distinctly *different* appearance, which will be described.

Orthokeratinized Epithelium

This type of epithelium (Fig. 3–8) consists of a basal layer (deepest), a prickle cell layer, a granular layer, and a keratinized layer.

The granular layer is located superficial to the prickle cell layer. The epithelial cells are flattened in shape and are filled with darkly staining *keratohyaline* granules. These granules consist of a chemical precursor of *keratin*. This layer is usually 2 to 4 cell layers thick. The most superficial cells in this layer contain the largest concentrations of the keratohyaline granules. The nuclei in those cells are somewhat flat and dark, showing signs of degeneration.

The *keratinized layer* is the superficial layer. There is an abrupt transition between the preceding granular layer and this layer. The cells in the keratinized layer have the shapes of flattened discs or *squames*. They are responsible for the name of this type of epithelium. The cells are no longer vital. *No nuclei* are present and most other organelles have been broken down as well. The contents of the keratohyaline granules have formed a complex with the tonofibrils. This complex is the *keratin* and this now fills the cells in this layer. The superficial-most cells become detached and are lost.

The thickness of this type of epithelium is variable. Areas of the body that are not normally subjected to a great deal of wear have a thin epithelium and a thin keratinized layer. Other areas have thicker epithelia. Especially thick epithelia and thick keratinized layers are found on the palm, sole and calluses.

Nonkeratinized Epithelium

The following layers are present in nonkeratinized epithelium (Fig. 3–9): (1) basal layer (deepest) and (2) prickle cell layer.

$\rightarrow$

Fig. 3–8. A, *Diagram of the characteristic superficial layers in orthokeratinized, stratified squamous epithelium. No detail is shown in the basal and prickle cell layers, which have been illustrated in Figure 3–7. The cells of the granular layer are flattened. As they move more superficially, they are filled gradually with keratohyaline granules. These darkly staining granules are responsible for the name of this layer. The superficial-most cells in this layer contain most granules. The keratinized layer is the most superficial layer of this type of epithelium. It consists of very flat cells, which have lost their organelles. Light microscopically no nuclei are visible in this layer. These nonvital cells are completely filled with keratin. The top cells of the keratinized layer are detached and lost. The bottom drawing is an enlarged detail, showing one cell from the granular layer and one cell from the keratinized layer. The transition between these 2 layers is as abrupt as the illustration shows.* B, *Histologic section of epidermis from a human fingertip. The various layers of keratinized, stratified squamous epithelium are illustrated. B = basal cell layer; P = prickle cell layer; G = granular layer; K = keratinized layer. Original magnification × 100.*

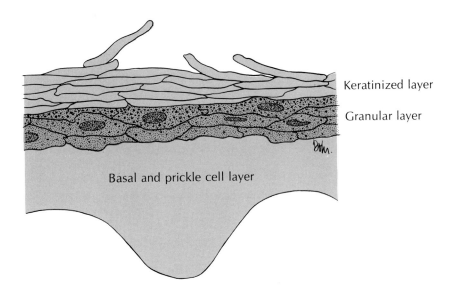

Keratinized layer

Granular layer

Basal and prickle cell layer

Keratin-filled cell

Keratohyaline granule

Nucleus

K
G
P
B

B

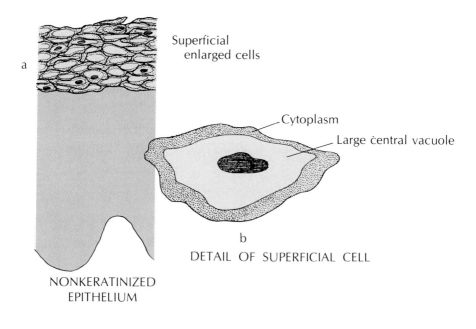

a

Superficial
enlarged cells

Cytoplasm

Large central vacuole

b
DETAIL OF SUPERFICIAL CELL

NONKERATINIZED
EPITHELIUM

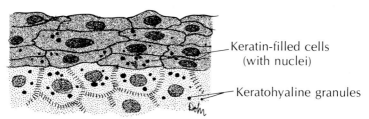

Keratin-filled cells
(with nuclei)

Keratohyaline granules

SUPERFICIAL CELLS IN PARAKERATINIZED EPITHELIUM

c

A

Fig. 3–9. A, *Diagram of a nonkeratinized, stratified squamous epithelium, a. No detail is shown in the basal and prickle cell layers, which have been illustrated in Figure 3–7. The superficial layer in this type of epithelium consists of gradually enlarging cells, with fluid accumulating in a centrally located space or vacuole. The nuclei remain present in these cells. The superficial-most cells are detached readily (see Fig. 3–6). In b, one of the superficial cells is shown. Its cytoplasm has been pushed toward the periphery of the cell, while the central part, fluid-filled in life, looks empty. The bottom diagram, c, shows the superficial layers of a parakeratinized, stratified squamous epithelium. In these layers the cells are gradually filled with keratin. However, few keratohyaline granules are formed, so that there is no distinct granular layer. In addition, the nuclei and other organelles remain present in the cytoplasm of the keratin-filled superficial-most cells. As in the other types of epithelium, the superficial cells are eventually lost.*

Fig. 3–9. (Cont'd) B, *A thick layer of nonkeratinizing, stratified squamous epithelium from the inside of a human lip, in histologic section. The superficial cells look empty and some have collapsed, owing to the loss of the central fluid during histologic tissue preparation. Original magnification × 100.* C, *Parakeratinized, stratified squamous epithelium from human attached gingiva, in histologic section. Compare this photograph with Fig. 3–8 B. In this epithelium no distinct granular layer is present, and the nuclei in the keratinized layer are still visible. Original magnification × 100.*

In this epithelium there are no further *distinctly* recognizable layers above the prickle cell layer. The cells undergo a gradual increase in size as they move closer to the surface of the epithelium. Because this increase in size is *not* accompanied by an increase in cytoplasmic organelles, the enlarged cells look *emptier*. Fluid-filled sacs, or *vacuoles*, form inside the cells and push the cytoplasm toward the cell membranes. In the largest superficial cells the cytoplasm remains only as a thin layer next to the cell membrane. The rest of these cells is filled with fluid.

There are several layers of such fluid-filled cells. They act as cushions and are firmly attached to each other, protecting the underlying tissues against mechanical damage.

Parakeratinized Epithelium

In this form of stratified squamous epithelium keratinization does occur, but without the widespread destruction of cellular organelles seen in orthokeratinization (Fig. 3–9, C).

As seen with the light microscope, parakeratinization differs from orthokeratinization in the following:

1. In parakeratinization a granular layer either does *not* form or remains indistinct. In either case some small keratohyaline granules may be seen in the cells closest to the keratinized layer.

2. The keratinized layer in parakeratinized epithelium contains cells in which the nuclei still may be visible. Parakeratinized cells are no longer vital, however, and their nuclei are shrunken and degenerated. These cells are gradually detached and lost.

Other Cell Types in Oral Epithelium

CLEAR CELLS. In addition to the epithelial cells, already described, the oral epithelium contains another group of cells, the so-called "clear cells." These cells have received their name because they have few or no desmosomal attachments to the surrounding epithelial cells. Following fixation, they shrink away from the surrounding cells and leave an empty, clear space around them.

Among the several types of clear cells, the most conspicuous are the *melanocytes*. These are the only type of clear cells we will describe here (Fig. 3–10).

Melanocytes are located in the basal layers of the oral epithelium, where they comprise approximately one-seventh of the total basal cell population. These cells have long extensions, protruding between the surrounding epithelial cells. They are responsible for the production of pigment, *melanin*. Melanin is present intracellularly in the form of specific granules. The granules, visible as intracellular brown dots in the light microscope, are transferred from the

Melanin granules

Fig. 3–10. Diagram of a melanocyte (darkly stippled), located between the basal cells of oral epithelium. Few or no desmosomes are present between these 2 different cell types. Melanin granules, produced by the melanocytes, are visible in the cytoplasm of these cells and are responsible for the pigmentation of the epithelium.

melanocytes to the basal epithelial cells. They are responsible for the brown color component of the oral mucosa.

In the skin, melanocytes are found in the basal layer of the epidermis. The differences in intensity of brown skin color between different racial groups does not seem to be due so much to the number of the melanocytes present as to the *rate of production* and *preservation* of the pigment granules.

If clinically visible pigmentation is present in the oral cavity, it is found in the attached gingiva (most frequently), the lips, the buccal mucosa and the soft palate. Pigmentation in the oral cavity does not *necessarily* coincide with pigmentation of the skin.

INFLAMMATORY CELLS. Certain cell types, commonly associated with inflammation, may transiently "immigrate" into the oral epithelium. This immigrant population includes lymphocytes, monocytes, neutrophilic granulocytes and, occasionally, mast cells. These cells do *not* commonly live and perpetuate themselves in the oral epithelium, as do the epithelial cells and the clear cells. These cell types will be discussed further in Chapters 4 and 6.

Interface Between Oral Epithelium and Lamina Propria

The interface between the oral epithelium and the underlying connective tissue is not smooth and straight, but corrugated. Where the two tissue types interdigitate, the epithelial extensions are called (epithelial) *rete pegs* and the connective tissue extensions *connective tissue papillae* (Fig. 3–11).

This corrugated arrangement is useful for 2 reasons:

1. It increases the surface area over which the two tissue types are in contact with each other. This in turn increases the *strength of the junction* between the two tissues. Areas that are subjected to a great deal of mechanical loading, such as the areas of the masticatory mucosa, have many thin, tall connective tissue papillae, interdigitating with many long epithelial rete pegs. The lining mucosa, on the other hand, has fewer and much shorter connective tissue papillae and wide, blunt epithelial extensions in between.

2. It decreases the distance between vascular supply and the epithelial cells. Epithelium does *not* have its own vascular supply. All blood vessels that carry the nutrients for the epithelial cells remain inside the connective tissue. Blood vessels in the connective tissue papillae can carry more nutrients closer to more epithelial cells than can blood vessels that are located underneath a straight epithelium-connective tissue interface (Fig. 3–12).

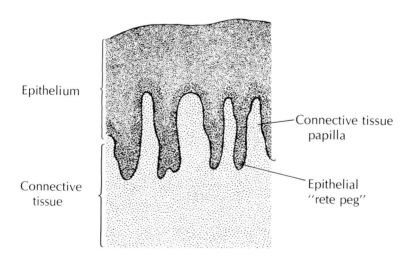

Epithelium

Connective tissue papilla

Epithelial "rete peg"

Connective tissue

Fig. 3–11. Diagram of a corrugated interface between epithelium and underlying connective tissue. Epithelial "rete pegs" alternate with connective tissue papillae.

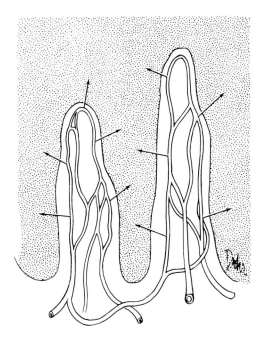

Blood vessels in
connective tissue papillae

Fig. 3–12. Epithelium does not have its own blood vessels. A rich blood vessel supply in the tall connective tissue papillae, penetrating deeply into the epithelium thickness, is capable of supplying many epithelial cells over short distances (arrows).

Basement Membrane at the Epithelium-Connective Tissue Interface

Between the basal cell layer of the oral epithelium and the underlying connective tissue, a sheet-like border structure is present: the *basement membrane* (Fig. 3–13).

The basement membrane is a noncellular structure, produced in part by connective tissue cells, in part by the basal epithelial cells. In the light microscope this structure is barely visible, having a thickness of only 1 to 2 μm. In the electron microscope more details are visible within the basement membrane.

The basement membrane is composed of *two* layers or *laminae.* Adjacent to the epithelial cells a thin, amorphous layer (20 to 70 nm

Basement membrane

Basement membrane { Basal lamina

Reticular lamina

Fig. 3–13. Light-microscopic (top) and electron-microscopic (bottom) appearances of the basement membrane, which is found between epithelium and the underlying connective tissue. Light-microscopically, the basement membrane is a very delicate, band-like structure, which is barely visible. Electron-microscopically, the basement membrane consists of a thin, darkly staining basal lamina and a much wider reticular lamina. Hemidesmosomal attachments (visible with the electron microscope only) are present between the epithelial cells and the basal lamina, which is a noncellular surface.

thick) is present. It appears as a thin, dark line in electron micrographs and is called a *basal lamina*. Its precise chemical composition is still not completely known, but we know that it contains many carbohydrates. The basal lamina is produced by the basal epithelial cells. These cells attach themselves to this lamina with *hemidesmosomes* (Chap. 2).

The remainder of the basement membrane is called the *reticular lamina*. It is considerably thicker than the basal lamina. The reticular lamina consists mainly of fibrous proteins *(reticulin)* and is produced by the connective tissue cells (Chap. 4).

Specialized Mucosa—The Tongue

The top surface of the tongue is covered with specialized mucosa. This mucosa is characterized by the presence of numerous *lingual papillae,* some of which have a *mechanical function* (remember that the tongue assists in the process of chewing), while others carry the specialized taste organs or *taste buds.*

The distribution of these papillae is best seen by inspection of your own tongue (in front of a mirror) and by comparison of your findings with Figure 3–14.

When inspecting the tongue, the part you see most readily is the *body* of the tongue. The body of the tongue comprises two-thirds of

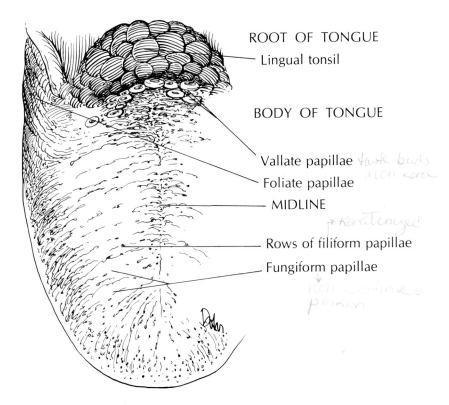

ROOT OF TONGUE
Lingual tonsil

BODY OF TONGUE

Vallate papillae
Foliate papillae
MIDLINE
Rows of filiform papillae
Fungiform papillae

Fig. 3–14. A fully extended human tongue. The body of the tongue makes up two thirds of its length, from the tip backward. It is covered with filiform papillae. Interspersed among these are occasional fungiform papillae. The root of the tongue makes up one third of its length. It is covered with tonsillar tissue. At the border between body and root of the tongue is a V-shaped row of vallate papillae. At about the same level, a few foliate papillae are present along the edges at the sides of the tongue.

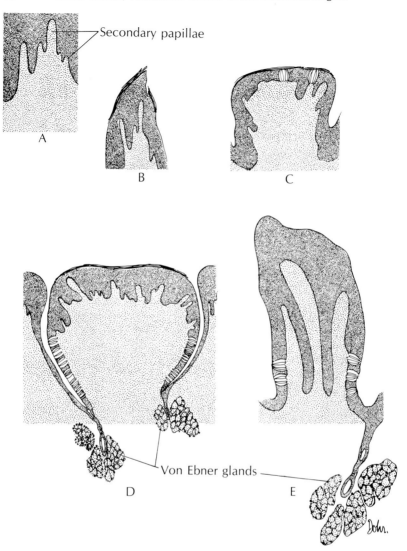

Fig. 3–15. Diagrams of the various lingual papillae. A, All lingual papillae have a connective tissue core or primary connective tissue papilla, illustrated here. Several smaller, conical secondary connective tissue papillae are present on top of the primary papilla. B, Filiform papilla. Conical in shape. The only lingual papilla without taste buds. Heavily keratinized epithelium. C, Fungiform papilla. Mushroom-shaped. Characterized by taste buds on the top surface of the papilla. The epithelium is very thin, with some keratinization. D, Vallate papilla. Mushroom-shaped. Characterized by a deep surrounding groove, into which some small salivary (von Ebner) glands open. Several taste buds are present on the sides of this papilla. E, Foliate papilla. Large, ridge-shaped. Deep grooves are present between neighboring papillae. Von Ebner glands open into these grooves. Taste buds are present on the side surfaces of these papillae.

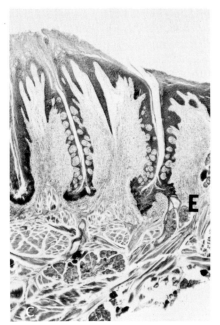

Fig. 3–16. A, *Filiform papillae (FL), heavily keratinized, and one fungiform papilla (FU) in a histologic section of a monkey tongue. A taste bud (arrow) is present on the top of the fungiform papilla. Original magnification × 12.5. B, Vallate papilla in a histologic section of a monkey tongue. Notice the deep groove around this papilla and the several taste buds (arrows) on its side. No von Ebner gland is visible in this particular section. Original magnification × 12.5. C, Three foliate papillae, separated by deep grooves, in a histologic section of a rabbit tongue. A von Ebner gland (E) opens into one of the grooves. Many taste buds are present on the sides of the papillae. Original magnification × 12.5.*

the tongue's length and lies horizontally in the oral cavity. Further back, near the throat, the tongue curves downward and becomes vertical. This vertical part of the tongue, comprising one-third of its length, is the *root* or *base* of the tongue. The body of the tongue carries the lingual papillae, while the base of the tongue is covered with tonsillar tissue (Chap. 6).

We distinguish 4 types of lingual papillae (Figs. 3–15 and 3–16): filiform papillae, fungiform papillae, vallate papillae, and foliate papillae. For the distribution of these papillae see Figure 3–14.

The *lingual papillae* consist of large, specialized connective tissue papillae, covered with orthokeratinized or parakeratinized stratified squamous epithelium. The basic structure of a (specialized) connective tissue papilla is that of a conical mountain (or a ridge, in the case of foliate papillae). This is the *primary papilla*. On top of the primary papilla several smaller, conical peaks or ridges are present. These are the *secondary papillae*.

FILIFORM PAPILLAE. These are the most abundantly present lingual papillae. They are spread over the entire surface of the body of the tongue and are covered with a thick layer of keratinized epithelium. These papillae have a purely *mechanical* function, and they are the only lingual papillae *without* taste buds.

FUNGIFORM PAPILLAE. These papillae are far less numerous than the filiform papillae. They are distributed among the filiform papillae and show as reddish dots on the surface of the tongue. They are shaped somewhat like mushrooms. A thin, keratinized epithelium covers their surfaces. The thinness of the epithelium allows the red of the blood vessels in the connective tissue papilla to show through. This is responsible for the red color of these papillae. On its *top* surface a fungiform papilla may carry one or several taste buds.

VALLATE PAPILLAE. These large papillae are located in a V-shaped groove at the border between body and base of the tongue. There are only 8 to 12 of these papillae. Their shape resembles that of the fungiform papillae, but the vallate papillae are sunk somewhat below the surface of the tongue, so that they are surrounded by a groove and a low, circular wall of oral mucosa. These papillae are covered with keratinized epithelium. Several taste buds are present on the vertical (side) surfaces of the papilla, facing the surrounding groove.

FOLIATE PAPILLAE. These papillae are 4 to 11 ridges, running parallel with each other on either side of the tongue, near the tongue base. These ridges may not easily be visible clinically. They are covered with keratinized epithelium and carry several taste buds on their sides.

The deepest parts of the grooves surrounding the vallate papillae and between adjacent foliate papillae contain the openings of ducts of special salivary glands, the *von Ebner glands*. Their serous saliva

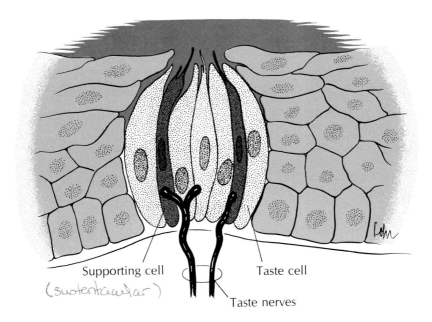

Supporting cell (suotentraular)   Taste cell

Taste nerves

Fig. 3–17. Diagram of a taste bud. The bud runs from the basement membrane to the top surface of the epithelium, where it is in contact with the saliva via a taste pore. Taste cells (which are specialized epithelial cells) with taste hairs and supporting cells (also specialized epithelial cells) are present in the taste bud. Delicate endings of taste nerves pass through the basement membrane and are in contact with the taste cells.

(Chap. 4) rinses the grooves continuously to enable the taste buds to perceive several different taste stimuli *in sequence.*

TASTE BUDS. Taste buds are barrel-shaped epithelial organs of special sense. While most of these organs are located on the lingual papillae, isolated taste buds may also be found on the soft palate and the wall of the pharynx.

Taste buds run from the basement membrane to the surface of the epithelium, across the entire epithelial thickness. The epithelial cells of the taste buds are tall and spindle-shaped. Some of these cells are *supporting cells,* surrounding and supporting the actual *taste cells.* The taste cells themselves have a *taste hair,* which protrudes into a surface opening of the epithelium, a *taste pore.* The taste pore provides a direct connection between the taste bud cells and the contents of the oral cavity. Molecules of materials to be tasted come to this taste pore (Fig. 3–17).

Stimuli of the taste sensations, perceived by the taste cells, are transferred to nerve endings that are in contact with the bases of the taste cells. These nerves carry the stimulus to the central nervous system, where the taste is *perceived* and *identified.*

SELECTED READING LIST

Arvidson, K.: Scanning electron microscopy of fungiform papillae of the tongue of man and monkey. Acta Otolaryngol., *81*:496, 1976.

Farbman, A.I.: Fine structure of the taste bud. J. Ultrastruct. Res., *12*:328, 1965.

Graziadei, P.P.C.: The ultrastructure of taste buds in mammals. In *Second Symposium on Oral Sensation and Perception.* Edited by J.F. Bosma, Springfield, Ill., Charles C Thomas, 1970.

Squier, C.A., and Meyer, J. (Eds.): *Current Concepts of the Histology of Oral Mucosa. Part I: The Oral Epithelium.* Springfield, Ill., Charles C Thomas, 1971.

Squier, C.A., Johnson, N.W., and Hopps, R.M.: *Human Oral Mucosa. Development, Structure and Function.* Oxford, Blackwell Scientific Publications, 1976.

Švejda, J., and Janota, M.: Scanning electron microscopy of the papillae foliatae of the human tongue. Oral Surg. Oral Med. Oral Path., *37*:208, 1974.

Švejda, J., and Škach, M.: The three-dimensional image of the lingual papillae. Folia Morphol., *22*:145, 1975.

Chapter *4*

ORAL MUCOSA—CONNECTIVE TISSUE PROPER

In the preceding chapter we learned that the lining of the oral cavity, the oral mucosa, consists of 2 tissue components—epithelium and connective tissue. The connective tissue component of the oral mucosa, called the *lamina propria,* itself consists of 2 layers: a *papillary layer,* comprising the connective tissue papillae and a thin common base, and a *dense fibrous layer,* comprising the bulk of the lamina propria. Between the oral mucosa and the underlying tissues (muscles for instance) there may be an intermediate layer of connective tissue, the *submucosa* (literally, *under the mucosa)* (Fig. 4–1).

The submucosa is structurally quite distinct from the lamina propria. It is a loose and delicate tissue. An oral surgeon uses this layer as a plane of dissection when placing the edge of the scalpel in the submucosa to lift the oral mucosa from the underlying tissues.

The submucosa is comparable, in structure and function, to the *hypodermis* beneath the skin. Hypodermic needles owe their name to the fact that they are used to inject substances into the hypodermis, the connective tissue layer underneath the skin. Similarly, for local anesthesia in the oral cavity, the submucosa is used for this purpose, *if it is present.* Some areas of the oral mucosa have little or

Fig. 4–1. *The oral mucosa is composed of oral epithelium (dark) and a layer of connective tissue proper: the lamina propria. The lamina propria is further subdivided in a papillary layer (lightly stippled), immediately underneath the epithelium, and a dense fibrous layer. Underneath the oral mucosa another connective tissue layer, the submucosa, may be present.*

no submucosa. (This is especially true in the case of masticatory mucosae: attached gingiva and mucosa of the hard palate.) If one attempts to give local anesthesia in such areas, the anesthetic will be able to infiltrate the dense tissue of the lamina propria only with difficulty, and this procedure is extremely painful. When possible, areas of the oral mucosa with a submucosa should be used instead (Fig. 4–2).

The tissues of the lamina propria and the submucosa are examples of *connective tissue proper*. This is only one tissue type within the larger group of *connective tissues*. Other connective tissues are

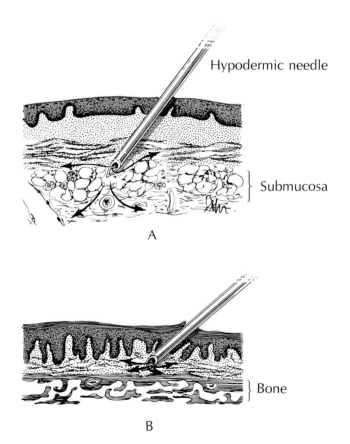

Fig. 4–2. When a thin hypodermic needle is used to inject substances underneath the oral mucosa, these substances will diffuse readily in the loose connective tissue of a submucosa, if present. This is the case in most areas of lining mucosae (A). Underneath masticatory mucosae a submucosa is usually absent. The lamina propria, which consists of dense connective tissue, is tied firmly to the underlying (bone) tissue (B). Injected substances do not diffuse readily and the resulting localized pressure is uncomfortable.

bone and cartilage, bone marrow, lymphoid tissue (tonsils and lymph nodes) and fat, as well as certain tissues of the tooth, i.e., pulp, dentin and cementum.

Collectively, connective tissues are a rather varied group. What these tissues have in *common* is that materials produced by the connective tissue cells assume a prominent role in the overall organization of these tissues. The various types of connective tissues *differ* in the nature of their cell products and in the proportions in which these products are present in the tissues.

CONNECTIVE TISSUE COMPONENTS

All connective tissues develop from embryonic connective tissue or *mesenchyme*. Mesenchyme consists of cells that produce intercellular material. As this intercellular material is deposited between them, the cells move apart, maintaining contact via small cell junctions, mostly desmosomes and tight junctions (Fig. 4–3).

The intercellular material generally consists of a fibrous matrix and a ground substance.

Fibrous Matrix

The fibrous matrix of a connective tissue is composed of some or all of the following: collagen fibers, reticulin fibers, elastic fibers, and oxytalan fibers.

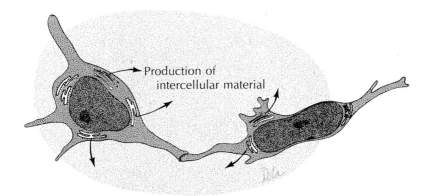

Production of
intercellular material

MESENCHYMAL CELLS

Fig. 4–3. Diagram of 2 mesenchymal cells. These cells have several long cell extensions, which are in junctional contact with similar extensions of neighboring mesenchymal cells. A few cisternae of rough endoplasmic reticulum, a medium Golgi complex and some mitochondria are present in the cytoplasm. Mesenchymal cells produce a water-rich intercellular material.

COLLAGEN FIBERS. Collagen is a protein. This means that collagen is produced in the rough endoplasmic reticulum of the connective tissue cell. It is then moved outside the cell via the Golgi complex, where some carbohydrates may be attached to it, and the secretory granules.

The structure of collagen and the various steps in its synthesis are beyond the scope of this book. Only a brief summary follows. The collagen product, released by the cell, consists of basic units. Each unit is composed of 3 long strands of proteins, twisted around each other. Some carbohydrates are attached to the surfaces of the unit. Outside the cells, many of these structural units, or *tropocollagen units,* undergo an organized assembly into collagen fibers.

Since the individual tropocollagen units are only 280 nm long and 1.4 nm wide, a large number of them is required to form the collagen fibers, which are visible with the light microscope (diameters: 1 to 15 μm), and the numbers needed to form an Achilles tendon (a structure consisting almost entirely of collagen) "staggers" the imagination.

The tropocollagen units are securely attached to each other by chemical bonds, and they line up in an orderly manner according to the *quarter stagger* model (Fig. 4–4). Fully assembled collagen fibers are capable of resisting *tension,* and when they are assembled, the fibers tend to form in a direction optimally suited to resist the tensions to which the tissue is subjected (Fig. 4–4).

RETICULIN FIBERS. During development of the organism, these fibers tend to appear first in connective tissue, but they gradually give way to increasing numbers of collagen fibers. Reticulin fibers are comparable to collagen fibers as far as their protein composition is concerned. While collagen fibers may become rather thick, reticulin fibers do not increase their diameters much beyond 1 μm.

Reticulin fibers tend to be associated with a considerably larger amount of carbohydrates than are collagen fibers. This accounts for the slightly different staining properties of the 2 fiber types. Reticulin fibers are formed predominantly in border areas between connective tissues and other tissues, for example, the reticular lamina of the basement membranes (Chap. 3).

ELASTIC FIBERS. Until recently, little was known about these fibers. They consist of long fibrous proteins of a different composition from those in collagen and are surrounded by a carbohydrate-rich mass. Certain components of this mass are specific for, and are only found in, elastic fibers.

Elastic fibers have diameters of 1 to 3 μm and they may be branched. Collagen fibers and reticulin fibers are *not* branched. Elastic fibers are responsible for the return of a connective tissue to its original arrangement following deformation of this tissue.

You may try this with the skin of your hand. Shift the skin over the underlying tissues as far as possible without hurting yourself. Then release. The resistance to this shifting movement came from the

Tropocollagen unit

Tropocollagen unit schematically

Tropocollagen units assembled in quarter stagger

Collagen fiber

Resists tension

Fig. 4–4. *The structural unit of collagen, tropocollagen, consists of 3 long protein strands, twisted around each other (top). For simplicity, the same tropocollagen unit has been redrawn even more schematically. The tropocollagen units align themselves in an orderly "quarter stagger" model, forming a collagen fiber. The bottom diagram illustrates that a collagen fiber is capable of resisting tension, imposed on it in the direction of its long axis (arrows).*

collagen fibers in the skin. The rapid recoil, following the release of this deformation, was due to the elastic fibers.

OXYTALAN FIBERS. These fibers closely resemble elastic fibers in morphology and chemical composition. However, there is one small chemical difference which makes it possible to stain these fibers selectively. It has been suggested that oxytalan fibers are immature elastic fibers.

Ground Substance

In addition to the fibrous matrix, connective tissue cells also produce a ground substance. Because this substance is frequently not visible in the light microscope, unless special stains are used, and is only barely visible in the electron microscope, it used to be called *amorphous* ground substance. The ground substance is, however, anything but amorphous. It consists of many large and highly organized carbohydrate chains attached to long protein cores.

The carbohydrates readily hold and bind water. They act somewhat as coils or springs, as the result of their particular chemical characteristics. The carbohydrates are responsible for the gelatinous

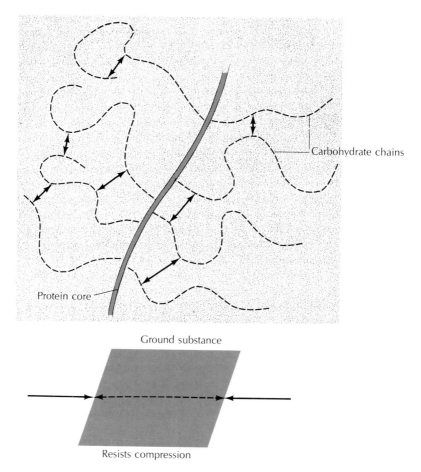

Fig. 4–5. *The structure of components of the ground substance is shown in this simplified diagram. Long carbohydrate chains are attached to a central protein core. The particular chemical nature of the carbohydrates prevents them from approaching each other too closely. Thus they act as molecular springs and are responsible for the resistance of ground substance to compressive loadings imposed on it from any direction (arrows in diagram).*

nature of the ground substance, which is highly resistant to *compression* (Fig. 4–5).

The preceding was a general introduction to the *intercellular* components of connective tissues. In the following section and in the next chapter we will discuss the specific details of certain types of connective tissues.

CONNECTIVE TISSUE PROPER

As does any other connective tissue, connective tissue proper consists of cells, fibrous matrix, and ground substance.

CELLS. The cells of connective tissue proper are fibroblasts, producers of the fibrous matrix and the ground substance, and other cell types for the maintenance and defense of the tissue.

FIBROUS MATRIX. The fibrous matrix consists of collagen, reticulin, elastin and oxytalan, with predominantly mechanical functions.

GROUND SUBSTANCE. The constituents of ground substance are carbohydrates and proteins, specific for connective tissue proper, with mechanical and biologic support functions, e.g., as pathways for metabolic products.

Organization of the Fibrous Matrix in Connective Tissue Proper

We noted before that both the lamina propria and the submucosa are examples of connective tissue proper, but it appears that even within this group further differences are possible. In the papillary layer of the lamina propria, as well as in the submucosa, the fibrous matrix is relatively delicate. It consists of thin collagen fibers, with relatively large, nonfibrous areas in between. In addition, this layer contains a fair amount of reticulin fibers. This type of connective tissue proper is called *loose connective tissue*. None of its 3 components (cells, fibrous matrix and ground substance) is particularly prominent.

The dense fibrous layer of the lamina propria is an example of *dense connective tissue*. In this tissue type the fibrous matrix has become the dominant component. Dense connective tissue consists predominantly of heavy, tightly packed, collagen fibers. You will remember that collagen is particularly well suited to resist *tension*. An understanding of the structure of this tissue leads to an understanding of its function. A dense connective tissue has a predominantly mechanical, tension-resisting function.

In the case of the dense fibrous layer of the lamina propria, the fibers are oriented in all directions, forming a 3-dimensional meshwork. This means that this dense connective tissue is capable of optimally resisting tension in *any* direction.

There are other dense connective tissues, in which the collagen fibers are all oriented in a flat plane, forming a 2-dimensional meshwork (the fasciae surrounding the muscles; the periosteum surrounding the bones). Such fibrous sheets resist tension, exerted largely in the plane in which the fibers are oriented.

In other dense connective tissues the collagen fibers are all oriented in only one direction (the tendon of a muscle). In such cases most tension is exerted, and resisted, in the direction in which the collagen fibers are oriented.

In *loose connective tissue* the collagen fibers and reticulin fibers run in all directions, but because of their delicate nature, they have only a minor mechanical function. The major function of a loose connective tissue is one of *biologic support*. It fills the spaces between organs and tissues and it carries blood vessels and nerves. In addition, it houses various types of cells engaged in the protection of the body. Thus it should *not* be surprising that the loose connective tissue of the papillary layer carries the rich vascular network that supplies the overlying epithelium, as well as the nerve terminals, that is, free nerve endings, which cross the basal lamina and enter the epithelium, and encapsulated nerve endings, which remain in the connective tissue.

The submucosa also carries a rich vascular network, as well as the major nerves and blood vessels, fat and glandular structures. Relatively smaller amounts of elastic fibers and oxytalan fibers are found in both types of connective tissue proper. They have mechanical functions.

Cells in Connective Tissue Proper

There are many types of cells, of varying and distinct functions, in connective tissue proper. A brief description of these cells will be given here. We distinguish 2 groups of cells: (1) cells that normally inhabit connective tissue (Fig. 4–6), and (2) wandering cells, normally circulating in blood, which enter the connective tissue by moving out of the blood vessels when needed.

Cells that *normally inhabit* connective tissue are almost all highly specialized and differentiated mesenchymal cells. Some *undifferentiated mesenchymal cells* may still remain in adult connective tissue. These cells are generally considered as a pool of reserve cells, which may differentiate at a later time, when needed.

FIBROBLASTS ("fiber-producers"). These cells consist of small cell bodies with several delicate cell extensions. Fibroblasts are responsible for the production of both fibrous matrix and ground substance. As might be expected, they all have the organelles necessary for the production of proteins and attachment of carbohydrates to the proteins.

In addition, these cells are also capable of breaking down their

FIBROBLAST

A

MACROPHAGE

B

MAST CELL

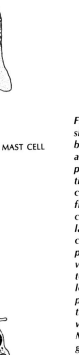

C

Fig. 4–6. A, Fibroblasts are spindle-shaped or star-shaped. They are responsible for the production of fibrous matrix and ground substance in connective tissue proper. ER = rough endoplasmic reticulum; G = Golgi complex; Vac = secretory vesicles; Tf = abundant tonofilaments (bundles of microfilaments in cytoplasm); Co = newly synthesized collagen fibers. B, Macrophage, or a histiocyte in which clear evidence of phagocytosis is present. PhV = phagocytic vacuoles, filled with various ingested materials; Ly = lysosomes; LD = lipid droplet; Pd = pseudopodium. An actively phagocytic cell may become mobile, and the small, transient pseudopodia are involved in the propagation of the cell. C, Mast cells are round to oval. The large granules in the cytoplasm have dense or crystalline (Cry) contents and are surrounded by a membrane. These granules contain the vasoactive substances heparin and histamine. Few organelles are present in these cells. (From Lentz, T. L.: Cell Fine Structure: An Atlas of Drawings of Whole-Cell Structure. Philadelphia, W.B. Saunders Co., 1971.)

MONOCYTE

POLYMORPHONUCLEAR LEUKOCYTE

LYMPHOCYTE

PLASMA CELL

Fig. 4-7. Wandering cells, which may be present in connective tissue proper. A, Monocytes have an abundant cytoplasm. An extensive Golgi complex and large numbers of lysosomes are indicative of the potential of this cell for digestive activities. When actively involved in phagocytosis, such cells become macrophages. B, A polymorphonuclear leukocyte is readily recognizable by its single, lobed nucleus, making it appear as if (in some sections) this cell had several nuclei. There are few organelles. Gly = several glycogen granules; SpG (specific granules) and AG (azurophilic granules) contain enzymes capable of digestion of phagocytosed materials. C, Lymphocytes have an almost spherical nucleus with a small indentation on one side. A narrow rim of cytoplasm surrounds the nucleus. Characteristically, large numbers of free ribosomes (R) are present in the cytoplasm. A few dense granules (Gr) are visible as well. D, A plasma cell has an ovoid, eccentrically placed nucleus, with a characteristic, cartwheel arrangement of chromatin. The cytoplasm contains an extensive rough endoplasmic reticulum and Golgi complex (active immunoglobulin synthesis). (From Lentz, T.L.: Cell Fine Structure: An Atlas of Drawings of Whole Cell Structure. Philadelphia, W.B. Saunders Co., 1971.)

62

own products. This enables them to continuously replace components of the intercellular materials, especially the rapidly "turned over" carbohydrate-rich substances.

HISTIOCYTES. These cells also have several cell extensions. They are located predominantly alongside the blood vessels. They are rich in lysosomes, which means that they are capable of digestive activities.

Ingestion (uptake) and digestion (intracellular breakdown) of extracellular matter is a process called *phagocytosis.* If a cell is involved in a great deal of phagocytosis, vacuoles filled with ingested materials become visible in its cytoplasm under the light microscope. When such clear evidence of phagocytosis is present, we no longer call such cells histiocytes, but *macrophages.*

MAST CELLS. These round-to-oval cells are found throughout the connective tissue, but by preference close to the blood vessels. Under the light microscope, many "grains" are visible in their cytoplasm. These are vesicles filled with 2 important substances, *heparin* and *histamine.* Heparin is an anticoagulant, a substance that prevents blood clotting. Histamine has a dilating (widening) effect on blood vessels. During an inflammation, mast cells discharge their contents in the ground substance. The resultant blood vessel reaction is one of the typical attributes of an inflammation, producing redness and later swelling of the tissues.

WANDERING CELLS. A number of cells normally carried in the blood stream may, when the need arises, move out of the blood vessels into the connective tissue proper (Fig. 4–7).

Some of these cells are capable of *digesting* harmful agents, or breakdown products (thus assisting the normal population of histiocytes); others may be involved in *immune responses* of the body,

Table 4–1. Wandering Cells of Connective Tissue Proper

Cell Type	Function	Where Found
1. *Monocytes*	Phagocytosis. When large amounts of extracellular materials are ingested, monocytes, like histiocytes, are called *macrophages*	Areas of inflammation
2. *Polymorphonuclear leukocytes* (neutrophils)	Destruction and ingestion of cells, bacteria and other harmful agents	Areas of chronic and acute inflammation
3. *Lymphocytes*	Participation in immune response, both humoral and cell-mediated	Areas of chronic and acute inflammation
4. *Plasma cells*	Production of immunoglobulins	Areas of chronic inflammation

or in the *destruction* of other cells. These cells, which are normal components of blood, will be noted briefly here and more extensively in Chapter 6.

FAT

Fat is a special type of connective tissue. It is composed of *fat cells*. They have differentiated from mesenchymal cells and their differentiation consists of an *intracellular* accumulation of fat (Fig. 4–8).

Frequently the cells are surrounded by delicate reticulin fibers. While fat cells may occur individually, they are more frequently assembled in groups, forming *fat tissue*. In the oral cavity some fat tissue is found in the submucosa of the hard palate, in the premolar region, making this a compressible area. Fat tissue may be present also in the submucosa, underneath the labial mucosa, and in the cheek, between cheek muscle and skin.

WHITE ADIPOSE CELL

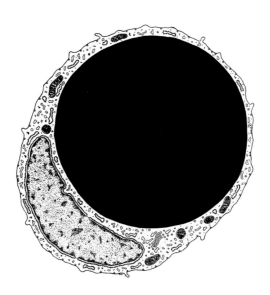

Fig. 4–8. *A white fat (adipose) cell is large. A central lipid droplet (dark) occupies most of the cell volume, and it is surrounded by a thin rim of cytoplasm. The nucleus is located in this peripheral cytoplasm and it is compressed into a crescent shape. A few organelles are scattered in the cytoplasm. (From Lentz, T.L.: Cell Fine Structure: An Atlas of Drawings of Whole Cell Structure. Philadelphia, W.B. Saunders Co., 1971.)*

SALIVARY GLANDS

Small (or *minor*) salivary glands are commonly found in the submucosa. They are present in the submucosa of the lips, the cheeks, parts of the hard palate (especially near the soft palate), the soft palate itself, the top surface of the tongue and the sublingual areas.

In addition to these minor salivary glands, we have 3 pairs of *major* salivary glands: the parotid glands, the submandibular glands, and the sublingual glands. The sublingual glands are located in the submucosa of the floor of the oral cavity. The 2 other pairs of major salivary glands are somewhat farther removed from the oral cavity. All glands, however, carry their products via their duct systems into the oral cavity.

Organization of Salivary Glands

Salivary glands are organs consisting of an *epithelial* and a *connective tissue proper* component.

The *epithelium* resembles a tree, in which the "base" is the opening of the duct leading into the oral cavity and the "leaves" are the parts where the production of the saliva begins. The intervening "twigs" and "branches" are components of the duct system, through which the secretion product is moved and modified, until it reaches the oral cavity as saliva (Fig. 4–9).

Dense connective tissue surrounds the entire epithelial tree, forming a connective tissue *capsule* around the gland. Around the individual epithelial components of the gland, within the capsule, less dense connective tissue is present. The connective tissue gives mechanical support to the epithelium and it carries the biologic support systems: the blood vessels and nerves.

Blood vessels and nerves have a branching pattern, similar to that of the epithelium, so that all epithelial components have rich blood and nerve supplies.

As a result of the branching pattern of the epithelial ductal tree, there is an uneven distribution of epithelial and connective tissue components in a salivary gland. The finer ducts and the "leaf" terminals form epithelium-rich *lobules,* in which most of the volume is occupied by epithelium (parenchyme) and a small part by delicate connective tissue (stroma), which surrounds the individual ducts and terminals.

Between the lobules are areas occupied by denser bands of connective tissue proper. These bands are called *septa*. They run convergingly from the peripheral capsule in the glandular mass and carry the larger epithelial ducts and the blood vessels and nerves, which will further branch inside the lobules.

The different components of the epithelial ductal tree have different functions and the epithelial cells have specialized accordingly. Before we discuss the various epithelial components of a salivary gland, review the discussion of intracellular organelles (Chap. 2) and of the classification of epithelia (Chap. 3).

Epithelial Ductal Tree

ACINUS. This is the "leaf" of the ductal tree of a salivary gland. Three-dimensionally an acinus is spherical. The epithelial cells forming the acinus are cuboidal and are arranged in a single layer. These are protein-carbohydrate producing cells and, therefore, have an abundant rough endoplasmic reticulum, Golgi complexes and secretory vesicles. Many secretory vesicles fill the slightly narrower top portion of the cell, where they will be released in the central opening or lumen.

An acinus may form 1 of 3 types of products. Depending on the product, one may have a serous acinus (producing a somewhat watery product, in which proteins are prominent), a mucous acinus (producing a more viscous product, in which large carbohydrates are prominent) or an intermediate mucoserous acinus. The distribution and proportions of the organelles in these different acinar cells vary with the nature of the product.

Most minor salivary glands have mixed, largely mucous acini. The exception is formed by the purely serous, minor salivary glands that are associated with vallate and foliate papillae on the tongue (von Ebner glands). Of the major salivary glands, the parotid has almost exclusively serous acini; the submandibular gland has both mucous and serous acini (mixed gland) and the sublingual gland has largely mucous and sero-mucous acini.

←

Fig. 4-9. A, Lobule of a developing salivary gland in a human fetus (second trimester of pregnancy). The tree-like arrangement of the darkly stained epithelium is clearly visible. Future saliva production will begin in the "leaves," and the saliva will be moved through the "twigs" and "branches" toward the oral cavity. Notice the rich blood supply (BV = blood vessels) in the lobule. C = developing connective tissue capsule; S = developing connective tissue septum. Original magnification × 40. B, Part of a connective tissue septum (S) and the parenchyma of an adjacent lobule (L) in a human parotid gland. A = acinus; St = striated duct; Se = excretory duct; F = fat cell. The tree-like structure of the epithelial component, while still existing, is no longer visible in a section of a mature salivary gland, owing to the increases in size and differentiation of the epithelial cells. Original magnification × 40.

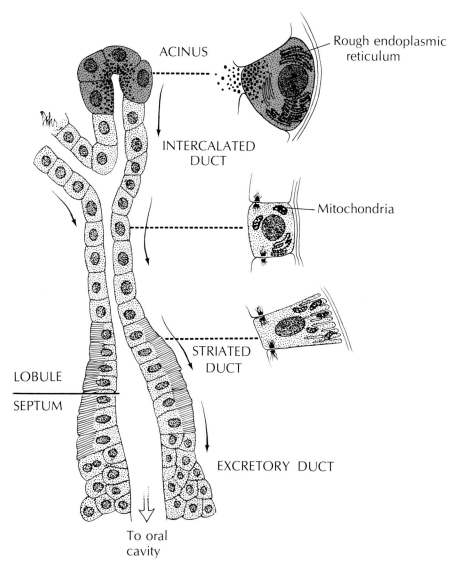

ACINUS

Rough endoplasmic reticulum

INTERCALATED DUCT

Mitochondria

STRIATED DUCT

LOBULE

SEPTUM

EXCRETORY DUCT

To oral cavity

Fig. 4–10. *Diagram of the epithelial components of a salivary gland. The arrows indicate the flow of the salivary product from acinus through intercalated, striated and excretory ducts toward the oral cavity. The acinus consists of a spherical mass of cells with a central lumen. Illustrated separately is a serous acinar cell, producing a protein-rich product. An extensive rough endoplasmic reticulum is present. A basal lamina surrounds the epithelial cells, separating them from the connective tissue stroma. Secretion of the product, via secretory vesicles, takes place into the central lumen of the acinus. The intercalated duct cells (one is illustrated separately) are cuboidal cells, separated from the surrounding connective tissue stroma by a basal lamina. Tight junctions and desmosomes are present adjacent to the lumen. A similar arrangement of tight junctions, desmosomes and basal lamina is found in the striated duct. Illustrated separately is a columnar striated duct cell, showing the rows of mitochondria between the basal membrane folds. The excretory duct is composed of transitional forms between a simple columnar epithelium (near the striated duct) and stratified squamous epithelium, near the oral mucosa. Part of the striated duct and the entire excretory duct are located in a connective tissue septum. The remainder of the ducts and the acini are located in a lobule.*

DUCTAL SYSTEM. Once it is secreted, the product moves from the lumen of the acinus into the lumen of the *intercalated duct*. This duct is a hollow tube, lined by a single layer of small, cuboidal, epithelial cells. The precise function of this duct is unknown. From the intercalated duct, the product moves next into the *striated duct*. This duct is a hollow tube, lined by a single layer of tall, columnar, epithelial cells. These cells, which show light microscopically a series of stripes in their bases (hence the name: striated), are involved in a substantial modification of the salivary product. Sodium ions, chloride ions and water are removed from the product and moved back, across the cells, into the blood. Simultaneously, potassium ions are taken out of the blood and added to the salivary product in the lumen of the striated duct.

Under the electron microscope, rows of mitochondria are found between deep folds of the basal cell membranes of these cells (under the light microscope these rows of mitochondria are visible as stripes). This arrangement supplies the energy to pump ions across the cells.

Acinar and ductal cells are firmly attached to each other, near their luminal surfaces, by tight junctions and complexes of junctions.

From the striated duct the salivary product moves into the *excretory duct*. This type of duct is the only component of the epithelial ductal tree, which is located entirely in a connective tissue septum (Fig. 4–10). All other components are located completely or partially inside the lobules. This duct forms a hollow tube, and its epithelial lining shows all transitional forms between a single-layered columnar epithelium (near the striated duct) and a stratified squamous epithelium (nonkeratinized, near the oral epithelium). This duct carries the saliva into the oral cavity.

Clinically, the location of the *major* salivary glands frequently can be identified by spurts of saliva coming from the openings of the excretory ducts underneath the tongue and on the cheek, near the upper molars. Multiple openings of ducts of the *minor* salivary glands, especially at the border between the hard and the soft palate, may cause salivary discharge when you take an impression of the upper jaw.

VARIATIONS IN THE STRUCTURE OF THE ORAL MUCOSA

As we have seen, there are 3 types of oral mucosa: lining mucosa, masticatory mucosa and specialized mucosa. While all lining and masticatory mucosae each have certain general characteristics (Chap. 3), there are some *regional differences*. A summary of the major differences is given in Tables 4–2, 4–3, and 4–4.

Table 4–2. Lining Mucosa

	Epithelium Nonkeratinized, stratified squamous	Lamina propria Papillary layer has short papillae	Submucosa Usually present
General characteristics			
Differences			
Lip and cheek	Very thick (500 μm)	Irregular papillae Dense fibrous layer contains collagen and some elastic fibers Rich vascular supply	Contains fat and minor salivary glands, mostly mucous in nature Firm attachment between lamina propria and connective tissue covering of muscles
Alveolar mucosa	Thin (app. 150 μm)	Papillae sometimes absent Many elastic fibers Rich vascular supply, running close to surface (clinically: appears red)	Loose connective tissue with many elastic fibers Minor salivary glands of mixed, mostly mucous, nature
Floor of mouth	Very thin (app. 100 μm)	Broad papillae Extensive vascular supply	Loose connective tissue with fat and sublingual glands
Undersurface of the tongue	Thin (app. 150 μm)	Thin, with numerous papillae Some elastic fibers A few minor salivary glands, mostly mucous and mixed	Absent The lamina propria is bound directly to the connective tissue, covering the tongue muscles
Soft palate	Thin (app. 150 μm)	Thick, with numerous papillae Elastic fibers form a distinct elastic lamina	Loose connective tissue with numerous minor salivary glands, mucous in nature

An immediate clinical application of some of these characteristics is the administration of certain drugs, such as nitroglycerin, to a patient with heart disease. The tablet is placed on the mucosa of the floor of the mouth, underneath the tongue. The drug is readily absorbed through the thin epithelium, entering rapidly the extensive blood supply in the underlying lamina propria. In this way the drug becomes effective in a brief period of time.

Adapted from Squier et al. 1976.

Table 4–3. Masticatory Mucosa

	Epithelium	*Lamina propria*	*Submucosa*
General characteristics	Keratinized or parakeratinized, stratified squamous	Tall, narrow papillae Pronounced dense, connective tissue layer Moderate vascular supply	Only sporadically present
Differences Gingiva	Thick (app. 250 μm) Often stippled orange peel appearance	Extensive blood vessel loops in papillary layer	*Absent* Lamina propria is continuous with the fibrous covering of the underlying bone tissue
Hard palate	Thick. Surface thrown into transverse ridges (rugae)	Thick, especially in the rugae	Present *only* on the sides of the hard palate Contains fat in the premolar area Minor *salivary glands* in the molar area (mostly mucous) Elsewhere, the lamina propria is continuous with the fibrous covering of the underlying bone

An immediate *clinical* application of some of these characteristics is the *compressibility* of the mucosa of the hard palate in the areas containing fat or glandular tissue. These areas are used preferentially to support upper dentures or removable orthodontic appliances. When dentures or appliances rest on areas without submucosa (noncompressible), they cause pressure spots, extremely painful, on those surfaces of the mucosa.

Adapted from Squier et al. 1976.

Table 4–4. Specialized Mucosa

	Epithelium	Lamina propria	Submucosa
Top surface of the tongue *only*	Thick, keratinized, stratified squamous	Distinct, specialized papillae	*Absent*
	Some nonkeratinized areas	Rich innervation, especially near taste buds	The lamina propria is continuous with the fibrous covering of the tongue muscles
	Specialized surfaces of lingual papillae: taste buds	Tonsillar tissue is present near the base or root of the tongue	
		There are many minor salivary glands	
		They are predominantly mucous or mixed, except near vallate and foliate papillae, where they are exclusively serous (Von Ebner glands)	

Adapted from Squier et al. 1976.

SELECTED READING LIST

Gordon, S., and Cohn, Z.A.: The macrophage. Int. Rev. Cytol., 36:171, 1974.

Lentz, T.: Cell Fine Structure. An Atlas of Drawings of Whole Cell Structure. Philadelphia, W.B. Saunders Co., 1971.

Ross, R., and Bornstein, P.: Elastic fibers in the body. Sci. Am., 224:44, 1971.

Schubert, M., and Hamerman, D.: A Primer on Connective Tissue Biochemistry. Philadelphia, Lea & Febiger, 1968.

Squier, C.A., and Meyer, J.: Current Concepts of the Histology of Oral Mucosa. Part II: The Connective Tissue of Oral Mucosa. Springfield, Ill., Charles C Thomas, 1971.

Squier, C. A., Johnson, N. W., and Hopps, R.M.: Human Oral Mucosa. Development, Structure and Function. Oxford, Blackwell Scientific Publications, 1976.

Weinstock, M., and Leblond, C.P.: Formation of collagen. Fed. Proc., 33:1205, 1974.

Young, J.A., and van Lennep, E.W.: Gross Anatomy. Microscopic anatomy. In The Morphology of Salivary Glands. New York, Academic Press, 1978.

Chapter 5

CONNECTIVE TISSUES: CARTILAGE AND BONE

Cartilage and bone are both skeletal tissues. In clinical practice these tissues usually are not visible, since they are covered with skin, oral mucosa, other connective tissue or even muscle tissue. But an awareness of the skeletal tissues must be an integral part of any dental treatment. More directly, you will often encounter the images of one of these skeletal tissues: bone, on dental x-ray films (roentgenograms).

X rays are used to study the structure of the so-called "hard tissues": bone and dental tissues. Such tissues owe their hardness to the presence of a mineral salt in their fibrous matrix and ground substance. This mineral salt forms a barrier for x rays. Soft tissues allow x rays to pass through and hit an x-ray film, placed behind the tissues. Those parts of the film, which have been hit by x rays, become dark. Any light areas represent those parts of the film from which the x rays were barred. Such light areas show the shapes and differential degrees of hardness of the structures which stopped the x rays, in general bone and teeth.

The x ray films shown in Figure 5–1 serve to illustrate this point. Notice the dense, solid (white) band, representing the bone at the periphery of the jaw: this is called *compact bone*. The compact bone layers enclose an area, which contains only delicate bone spangs, or *trabeculae*. This is called *spongy bone*. Between the bone trabeculae a soft, specialized connective tissue is present: bone marrow.

Any absence or disruption of the normal patterns of compact and spongy bone are indicative of a disease process, such as an area of inflammation around the tip of a dental root, or advanced periodontal disease.

Bone and cartilage are both specialized types of connective tissue. While connective tissue proper has many different functions (see Chap. 4), which in part is illustrated by the variety of cell types in it, bone and cartilage are uniquely specialized for *support* functions. This means that the intercellular substance of these tissues has assumed important properties.

Fig. 5–1.   X-ray images of a human lower jaw. A, *Intact lower jaw. The second molar has been lost. Clearly visible within the jaw is the bony canal (arrow), which contains the nerves and the blood supply to the teeth and surrounding tissues. Notice that the peripheral parts of the jaw are lighter in the roentgenogram. This means that the bone in those parts is more compact than in the central regions.* B, *The same lower jaw as shown in* A. *The first molar and the first premolar have been removed, making the outlines of their bony sockets more clearly visible. The lower jaw has been cut into several sections (a through i).* C, *The cut sections of the lower jaw have been x-rayed individually, with their cut surfaces parallel to the x-ray film (turned 90 degrees from their orientation shown in* B). *The peripheral compact bone and the central spongy bone are clearly shown. In b through g the dark openings of the cross-sectioned bony canal are visible.*

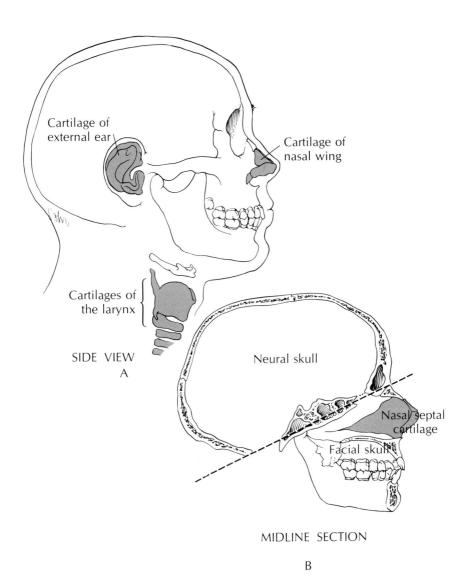

Cartilage of external ear

Cartilage of nasal wing

Cartilages of the larynx

SIDE VIEW

A

Neural skull

Nasal septal cartilage

Facial skull

MIDLINE SECTION

B

Fig. 5–2. Side view, A, and midline section, B, of a human skull, showing the bony components and the cartilaginous parts. In the adult, cartilage is found in the ear, the nose and the larynx.

Cartilage is a resilient "bouncy" tissue. It is uniquely suited to resist *compression*. It should be clear, from the previous chapter, that cartilage has this property because of an overwhelming amount of *ground substance*, which dominates the intercellular substance.

Bone is a rigid tissue, capable both of resisting *tension* and of giving *support*. It has these properties because of a large amount of *collagen fibers* and because of its impregnation with the mineral calcium salt: *hydroxyapatite*. This calcium salt is responsible for the images of bones on x ray films, since calcium salts do not allow the x rays to pass through.

While bone is more important for the dental health professional, cartilage is found in several parts of the body that surround the oral cavity (Fig. 5–2). Furthermore, a knowledge of cartilage tissue is of use in understanding bone tissue. For this reason, we will start here with a description of cartilage.

CARTILAGE

Cartilage has the 3 components that are generally found in all connective tissues: *cells* (chondroblasts, chondrocytes), *fibrous matrix* (collagen, in special cases elastin as well), and *ground substance* (specific long carbohydrate chains, bound to protein). Of these 3 components the ground substance is the dominant one.

CELLS. Cartilage cells differentiate from the common forerunners of connective tissue cells: the mesenchymal cells. During their differentiation, these cells move closer together than the mesenchymal cells, which will form connective tissue proper. This *mesenchymal condensation* takes place before the cells start producing the fibrous matrix and ground substance characteristic for cartilage (Fig. 5–3; review synthetic activities of a cell, Chap. 2).

FIBROUS MATRIX. The fibrous matrix of cartilage consists of a sparse network of delicate collagen fibers. This collagen has the same *basic* characteristics as the collagen in connective tissue proper, but with a few, relatively minor, chemical differences, which make this a specifically cartilaginous collagen.

GROUND SUBSTANCE. The ground substance of cartilage consists of large carbohydrate chains, attached complexly to protein "backbones." The nature of these carbohydrate chains and their relative proportions are specific for cartilage, and they largely determine the nature of this tissue. Such enormous amounts of ground substance are formed that the fibrous matrix is completely masked and is not visible with conventional light microscopic techniques.

With the production of these intercellular materials, the cells, *chondroblasts,* become eventually enclosed by their own products. When this happens, they lose their contacts with the surrounding cells and come to lie in isolation in a small space or *lacuna* inside

Fig. 5-3. *Histologic section through a mesenchymal condensation* (arrow) *in a 5½-week-old human embryo. These condensed mesenchymal cells will soon start producing cartilage. Other mesenchymal condensations are present as well. Some of these will develop further into muscles, others into bone tissue. Original magnification × 100.*

Fig. 5-4. *Histologic section through a cartilage structure in a newborn. The cartilage ground substance is the dominant component of this tissue, masking the fibrous matrix completely. Chondrocytes, fully enclosed within lacunae, are present throughout the tissue. Some are grouped in nest-like arrangements (N). At the periphery of the cartilage, the cell-rich zone of the perichondrium is visible. This zone contains chondroblasts, some of which are partially enclosed in lacunae* (arrow), *in the process of becoming chondrocytes. Original magnification × 100.*

the intercellular substance. Such *enclosed* cells are called *chondro-cytes.*

They slow down considerably in their synthetic activities (although not completely); there is still turnover of the ground substance and some of the components of the fibrous matrix. The chondrocytes are responsible for this continued, slower, synthetic activity.

Early cartilage resembles a gelatinous mass, in which a number of chondrocytes are embedded. On the outside surface of this mass a layer of chondroblasts remains present. These cells continue the production of new intercellular material, which is deposited at the circumference of the cartilage. Occasionally, one of the chondroblasts is enclosed and becomes a new chondrocyte (Fig. 5–4).

Cartilage Growth

Once a chondrocyte is enclosed in a lacuna, it is still able to undergo some cell division or mitosis. The two resulting daughter cells utilize the somewhat liquid nature of the intercellular substance to "float apart," while producing a little more matrix in the process. As a result of the mitosis and of the synthetic activity, the daughter cells are found in *"cell nests,"* groups of 2, 3 or 4 chondrocytes, close enough to show their common descent, but enclosed in separate, individual lacunae.

The processes of mitosis and of production of new intercellular substance by the chondrocytes lead to an increase of the overall size of the cartilage mass. This is called *interstitial growth.*

In addition to this, the cartilage mass has a second growth mechanism: the increase in size resulting from new cartilage formation on its outside surface by the layer of chondroblasts. This is called *appositional growth* (Fig. 5–5).

With further development, the cartilage mass becomes more and more organized. The cartilage, with its peripheral layer of chondroblasts, becomes completely surrounded by a dense fibrous connective tissue layer. This layer, together with the layer of chondroblasts, is called a *perichondrium* (literally, around the cartilage).

The perichondrium, in addition to its mechanical functions as the site of attachment for muscles and as the outer membrane defining the shape of the cartilage mass, also contains most of the blood vessels, supplying the nutriments for the cartilage cells. The liquid nature of the intercellular substance of cartilage allows easy movement *(diffusion)* of gases and nutrients *to* the chondrocytes and of metabolic waste products *away* from the chondrocytes. Thus, there is relatively little need for blood vessels to be present *inside* the cartilage tissue. Cartilage is sometimes called an *avascular* tissue (no blood vessels at all), but this is only true for small cartilage

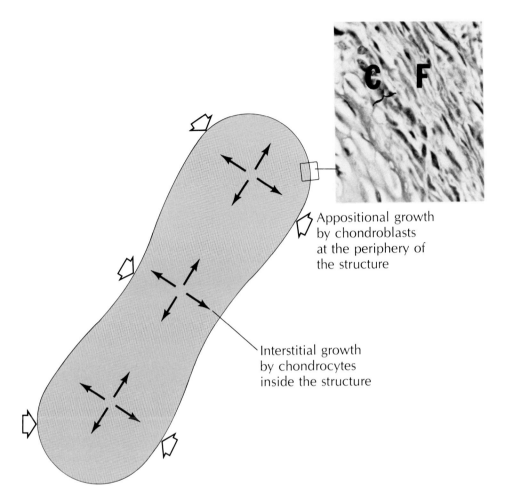

GROWTH OF A CARTILAGINOUS STRUCTURE

Fig. 5-5.   Diagram of a cartilage structure. The small arrows within the structure indicate that it can increase its size "from within" by mitoses of the chondrocytes and production of new intercellular substance (interstitial growth). The larger, open arrows indicate the second mechanism of growth of a cartilage structure, by production of new cartilage "on the outside" (appositional growth). The chondroblasts in the inner layer of the perichondrium are responsible for the appositional growth. Insert, Histologic section showing the 2-layered structure of perichondrium in a human fetus. An inner layer, adjacent to the cartilage, is cell-rich (C) and contains the chondroblasts. The outer layer of the perichondrium consists of densely arranged collagen fibers (F). There are some collagen fibers in the inner layer and some cells in the outer layer, but the layers of the perichondrium are named after their dominant components. Original magnification ×125.

masses. Some blood vessels may run for some distance into *larger* masses of cartilage. We therefore prefer to call cartilage a *relatively avascular* tissue.

The cartilage tissue we have described up to this point is *hyaline cartilage*, one of 3 types of cartilage found in the human body. We distinguish hyaline cartilage, fibrous cartilage, and elastic cartilage.

HYALINE CARTILAGE is predominantly a compression-resistant tissue. Its intercellular substance is dominated by the ground substance, which masks the collagenous fibrous matrix. This "reinforced gelatin" type tissue is found in many areas of the body. In the head and neck region, hyaline cartilage is found in the skeleton of the nose, in the growing skull base, in the condylar head of the lower jaw and in the larynx.

All cartilages in the human body start out as hyaline cartilages, but depending on their specific locations and loading patterns, some cartilages may specialize further and become either fibrous or elastic cartilage.

FIBROUS CARTILAGE. In this type of cartilage, such large amounts of collagen fibers are added to the intercellular substance that the ground substance loses its relative prominence and the fibers are no longer masked, becoming visible with the light microscope. Microscopically, this tissue somewhat resembles tendon tissue, with the exception that the cells (chondrocytes) are enclosed in lacunae. Fibrous cartilage is found in areas that are subjected to combinations of compression and tension, such as the discs in the vertebral column. In the head, only the temporomandibular joint of an older individual may contain some fibrous cartilage.

ELASTIC CARTILAGE. Normally, few or no elastic fibers are found in cartilage, but sometimes such fibers are *added* to the intercellular substance in cartilages that are in need of elastic rebound, such as the external ear and the epiglottis. The elastic fibers form a delicate fibrous matrix. They are not seen with conventional light microscopy, unless they are made visible with a specific elastic stain.

BONE

Bone has the 3 components commonly found in connective tissues: *cells* (osteoblasts, osteocytes, osteoclasts), *fibrous matrix* (collagen fibers), and *ground substance* (long carbohydrate chains, attached to protein "backbones"). Of these 3, the fibrous matrix is the dominant component. *In addition,* the nature of bone tissue is determined, to a large extent, by the presence of calcium salts *(hydroxyapatite)* in its intercellular substance.

Biomechanically, bone is particularly well suited to resist tension and brief periods of compression. If placed under any prolonged compression, bone tissue will readily yield by disappearing (see discussion of bone resorption in this chapter).

Bone tissue has 2 principal functions: (1) it gives biomechanical support and protection to the associated tissues and organs; and (2) it serves as a large reservoir for calcium and phosphorus ions (hydroxyapatite is a calcium phosphate salt). Calcium and phosphorus ions are critical for the maintenance of life. To this end, these ions must be constantly present in the circulating blood, where their concentration levels have to be maintained within narrow limits—10 mg Ca/100 ml (dl) blood and 6 mg P/100 ml (dl) blood. If these concentrations drop, immediate endocrine action stimulates increased breakdown of bone to liberate more ions. If the concentrations become too high, a different kind of endocrine action slows down the breakdown of bone.

For an understanding of bone tissue, it is necessary to understand not only its mode of formation, but also its constant *remodeling* throughout life: breakdown of bone tissue *(resorption)* and new formation of bone *(deposition).* In healthy adults, about 4% of all bone tissue is broken down at any given time.

Bone tissue is formed by *osteoblasts,* differentiated mesenchymal cells, but despite this common denominator, bone may develop in one of 2 different ways:

1. *Intramembranous ossification.* Mesenchymal cells move closer together (mesenchymal condensation), differentiate into osteoblasts, and begin to produce the intercellular substance of bone directly.

2. *Endochondral ossification.* This is a process of bone formation with an intermediate stage. The future bone is preformed as a cartilage model. This is subsequently destroyed, and on its remains newly differentiated osteoblasts deposit bone tissue.

Figure 5–6 illustrates which parts of the bony skull are formed by intramembranous ossification and which by endochondral ossification. Without discussing each individual bone, it should be clear from this figure that the bones of the *cranial base,* between the neural skull and the facial skull, form by endochondral ossification, whereas the bones of the facial and neural skulls form largely by intramembranous ossification. Minor exceptions to this general rule are a small part of the nasal septum, the nasal conchae, and the articulating condylar head of the lower jaw, all of which form endochondrally.

Intramembranous Ossification

The initial stages of this process are similar to those of cartilage development. Mesenchymal cells move closer together into mesenchymal condensations, differentiate into *osteoblasts* and begin to produce the intercellular substance, characteristic for bone.

Bone formation involves one *additional* step, however: after

Fig. 5–6. Histologic section, near the midline, through the facial region of a human fetus in the second trimester of pregnancy. Intramembranous ossification (direct bone formation) is taking place in the lower jaw (LJ), upper jaw (UJ), and palate (P). Endochondral ossification (bone formation, with an intermediate cartilage stage) occurs in the skull base (SB). Original magnification × 2. (Courtesy the late Dr. E. Applebaum.)

some intercellular substance has been laid down by the osteoblasts, these cells now deposit calcium salts in it. The precise mechanism of this *calcification* process and the question as to which osteoblastic organelles are involved in it remain to be elucidated.

There is always a lag period between the time of intercellular substance production and the full calcification of the bone tissue. Because of this, there is always a narrow, uncalcified seam of bone (the *osteoid seam*) immediately underneath the osteoblasts. This seam represents the most recently formed fibrous matrix and ground substance (Fig. 5–7).

As in the case of cartilage, the earliest osteoblasts soon become surrounded by their own products, and they are enclosed in small spaces or *lacunae*. The enclosed cells are *osteocytes*. They differ from chondrocytes in 2 important aspects:

1. They do not become isolated like the chondrocytes, but retain desmosomal and tight junctional contacts with neighboring osteo-

Fig. 5–7. Histologic section, illustrating early intramembranous ossification in the upper jaw region. A delicate network of bone trabeculae alternates with a network of thin-walled blood vessels (BV). Osteoblasts (arrows) line the surfaces of the bone trabeculae. A thin band of uncalcified bone (osteoid) intervenes between osteoblasts and calcified bone. A few cells have become trapped in lacunae inside the bone substance. These cells (osteocytes) have slowed down their synthetic activities considerably. Original magnification × 125.

Fig. 5–8. Histologic section through one half of the upper jaw region of a human fetus in the second trimester of pregnancy. This section shows a fundamental difference in appearance between developing cartilage and bone tissues. The cartilage of the nasal frame (NF) is one solid, homogeneous mass, somewhat thickened at the edges. The bone of the developing upper jaw (UJ) and palate consists of a delicate network of bone trabeculae, which alternates with a network of blood vessels (the latter are not visible at this magnification). Original magnification × 2. (Courtesy the late Dr. E. Applebaum.)

cytes and osteoblasts. The cell processes, which make these contacts, are thin and are located inside narrow bony channels or *canaliculi*, which run from lacuna to lacuna and from lacuna to the outside surface of the bone mass. The osteocytic lacunae, therefore, do not have a smooth, rounded outline like that of the chondrocytic lacunae. Instead, they are spider-shaped.

2. They are surrounded by a *calcified* intercellular substance. This means that there is no room for further cell divisions and therefore the bone *cannot* grow by interstitial growth.

Furthermore, the calcified matrix is an effective barrier, preventing diffusion of nutrients, gases and waste products. Instead, all this transport has to utilize the system of canaliculi between the outside of the bone and the individual lacunae. This type of transport can only take place over a limited distance (about 200 μm), which is the farthest distance an osteocyte may be removed from a blood vessel. Thus, while cartilage is relatively avascular, bone tissue is vascular.

Because of the high metabolic activities of osteoblasts and osteocytes, *and* because blood vessels are needed in the proximity of the osteocytes, the entire appearance of a developing bone is from the start different from that of a developing cartilage structure (Fig. 5–8).

A cartilage structure develops as one solid, homogeneous mass. A bony structure develops as a loose network of bone trabeculae, associated with a network of blood vessels. Each bone trabecula consists of a mass of calcified bone substance with osteocytes in their lacunae. Along the periphery of the trabecula is a layer of osteoblasts. Each individual bone trabecula grows by *appositional* growth only. Interstitial growth is not possible in bone tissue.

In time, a *periosteum* develops, surrounding the entire complex of small bone trabeculae and its blood vessel network. It consists, as does a perichondrium, of a dense fibrous layer on the outside and an inner cellular (osteoblasts) layer, next to the outermost surfaces

$\rightarrow$

Fig. 5–9. A, *The trabecular network of spongy woven bone in a histologic section through the lower jaw of a human fetus. Each trabecula is lined with osteoblasts. Continued bone deposition by these cells will make the individual trabeculae thicker and thus the bone as a whole more compact. A fibrous layer of periosteum (P) is forming at the periphery of the entire complex of bone trabeculae. This periosteum outlines the shape of the future bone. Original magnification × 40. B, Compact lamellar bone at the periphery of the lower jaw of an adult. The only interruptions in this bone mass are the channels (arrows) carrying the blood supply of the bone cells in the osteocytic lacunae. This compact bone was formed, in part, as the result of bone deposition around the individual trabeculae, making the bone more compact, and, in part, as the result of deposition of lamellar bone by the osteoblasts in the periosteum. The dark lines in the bone are arrest lines (A) and reversal lines (R), evidence of the constant remodeling of bone tissue. Original magnification × 40.*

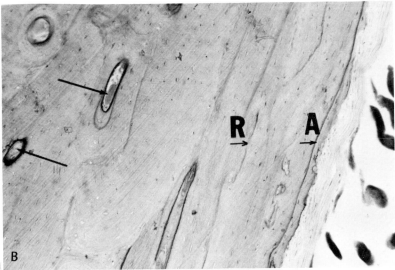

of the bone. This periosteal layer of osteoblasts is responsible for the increase in external dimensions of the bone complex by appositional growth.

In summary, the osteoblastic activities lead to (1) an increase in the *external* dimensions of the bone, if the osteoblasts are located in the periosteum; and (2) an increase in the size of the smaller components of the bone, the bone trabeculae, if the osteoblasts are located at their periphery. This increase in size of the bone trabeculae does *not* make the bone as a whole bigger, just more solid (Fig. 5–9).

Compact and Spongy Bone; Woven and Lamellar Bone

When a bone is cut open and inspected with the unaided eye or studied on the x-ray film, it is possible to distinguish between *compact* and *spongy bone.* This is a gross distinction.

At the microscopic level, we distinguish 2 types of bone tissue, *woven* and *lamellar* bone. This distinction is based on the organization of the fibrous matrix within the tissue.

WOVEN, SPONGY BONE. The earliest formed bone has a fibrous matrix, which consists of a 3-dimensional collagenous network. No distinct preferential orientation of these collagen fibers is demonstrable. Such bone is called woven bone. Woven bone is usually *spongy* (trabecular).

LAMELLAR BONE. When the bone becomes functionally loaded, it is in need of a better engineering design, and the woven bone is gradually replaced by *lamellar bone.* Lamellar bone is somewhat comparable to plywood. It consists of a series of thin sheets, or *lamellae,* 4 to 7 μm wide. Within each sheet the collagen fibers run parallel to each other, but in a different direction from that of the collagen fibers in the adjacent sheets. This arrangement gives the mature bone tissue an optimal ability to withstand the varieties of loading patterns imposed on it.

COMPACT, LAMELLAR BONE. At the periphery of a bone, such as the lower jaw, the osteoblasts of the periosteum produce a series of lamellae, parallel to each other and to the bone surface. These lamellae form a dense, *compact* layer of bone. However, the thickness of this layer is limited by the nutritional needs of the osteocytes. This need may be solved in different ways (Fig. 5–10): (1) inclusion of a blood vessel from the surrounding periosteum; and (2) breakdown of some of the older lamellar bone and outgrowth of a branch of a neighboring blood vessel in this newly created space. This blood vessel is subsequently surrounded by new bone.

Bone that is deposited around existing blood vessels is also lamellar bone, but as the result of its particular location, this bone

Periosteum

Blood vessel

Osteocytic lacuna

B

Primary osteon

Periosteum

A

Secondary
osteon

Blood vessel
surrounded by
newly formed bone

C

Fig. 5–10. **A,** *Highly schematic illustration of lamellar bone, immediately adjacent to periosteum. Osteoblasts comprise the inner layer of the periosteum, between the dense fibrous outer layer and the bone lamellae. Three lamellae are illustrated, with some (dark) osteocytic lacunae. The collagen fiber direction in the bone of the individual lamellae is indicated by parallel lines. Note that, within each lamella, all collagen fibers run parallel to each other, but in a different direction than the collagen fibers in adjacent lamellae.* **B,** *Enclosure of a periosteal blood vessel and formation of a primary osteon around it. The periosteal osteoblasts produce layer upon layer of bone lamellae, parallel to the outer bone surface. Occasionally, a blood vessel of the periosteum is left behind in the developing bone. Osteoblasts line the surface of the hollow space around the blood vessel and these cells produce concentric bone lamellae, forming a primary osteon around the blood vessel.* **C,** *Formation of secondary osteons. If continued bone lamella production by periosteal osteoblasts is not accompanied by occasional blood vessel inclusion, some of the older lamellar bone will be broken down. This older bone is located more centrally (deeper). After the breakdown, branches of neighboring blood vessels grow out into this newly established space. Around each of these blood vessel branches new, concentric bone lamellae are deposited and a secondary osteon is formed. A secondary osteon differs from a primary osteon in that a secondary osteon has a scalloped, not a smooth, outer surface. The surface is scalloped because bone breakdown precedes the formation of a secondary osteon. The scalloped edge reflects the final resorption surface with resorption lacunae–the "last bites," as it were, into the bone tissue, during the process of breakdown.*

forms a hollow cylinder of *concentric lamellae,* an *osteon.* Owing to its arrangement, an osteon has particular biomechanical properties that make it well suited to resist a large variety of loading patterns, such as those applied to the long bones of the limbs, where they are found in large numbers.

In the flat bones of the skull, osteons are not as numerous. The predominant pattern of compact bone in these bones is one of flat, parallel lamellae.

SPONGY, LAMELLAR BONE. The trabeculae in the spongy bone areas of the jaws consist of lamellar bone as well. Just as with compact bone, the spongy bone undergoes constant remodeling. The orientation of the trabeculae is a good indication of the loading patterns imposed on the bone. In general, the trabeculae are oriented in 2 main directions: one is parallel with the principal loading direction; the other is at right angles with the first. If the loading pattern changes, bone remodeling follows, adjusting the size and/or orientations of the bone trabeculae to the new condition.

Between the bone trabeculae *bone marrow* may be found. This specialized connective tissue consists of fat and/or blood-forming cells. A characteristic of spongy bone is that the overall volume of the marrow is greater than that of the bone mass.

Bone Resorption

Several times in the foregoing discussion the concept of *bone breakdown* or *resorption* has been mentioned. Bone resorption may take place for 2 different reasons:

1. Adaptation of the internal and/or external structure of the bone to altered loading conditions. In this case resorption is usually a *localized* process.

2. Liberation of calcium and phosphorus ions in response to endocrine activity. In this case resorption is a *general* process throughout the body.

Bone resorption involves two activities, dissolution of the bone salts (by acid from the lysosomes, released outside the cell) and breakdown of the intercellular bone substance (a digestive activity, also involving lysosomes). While osteoblasts and osteocytes are moderately capable of some bone resorption, the serious resorption is done by a special cell type, which differentiates when the need arises and disappears again when the job is done.

This cell is the *osteoclast.* It forms by *fusion* of several cells (of mesenchymal origin). Because of this, the osteoclast is *large* and it contains several nuclei (usually 4 to 10). It has a large number of lysosomes for its digestive activities (Fig. 5–11).

The osteoclast moves next to the bone surface, which needs to be broken down (see the 2 possible configurations in Fig. 5–12) and

OSTEOCLAST

Fig. 5–11.   *Diagram illustrating the ultrastructure of part of an osteoclast. The dark mass in the lower left hand corner is the bone, which is about to be resorbed. In the osteoclast parts of 3 nuclei are visible. The cell contains an extensive Golgi complex (G), numerous mitochondria and lysosomes. A small section of the cell membrane lies flat against the surface of the bone (arrow), and the adjacent cytoplasm is very clear. This is the region of the seal, which completely surrounds the digesting surface of the osteoclast. That part of the osteoclast's membrane, which is engaged in bone resorption (digestive activity), is thrown into large folds (ruffled border). This substantially increases the surface area of the cell. Gr = granules (lysosomal). (From Lentz, T. L.: Cell Fine Structure. An Atlas of Drawings of Whole Cell Structure. Philadelphia, W.B. Saunders, 1971.)*

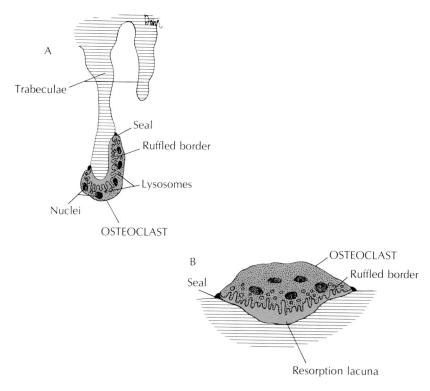

Fig. 5–12. *Diagrams of 2 possible configurations of osteoclasts and bone surface. A, An osteoclast is perched on the tip of a bone trabecula, partially surrounding it. The resorption will result in a reduction in length of the trabecula. B, An osteoclast is located on a flat surface of bone. In this case resorption will result in the illustrated depression (or resorption lacuna) in the bone surface. Notice, in both cells, the seal, which surrounds the ruffled border area and localizes the resorption process. Multiple nuclei and lysosomes are illustrated.*

seals off the area with a seal reminiscent of a suction cup. In this way the cell can discharge acid and lysosomal enzymes without harming other parts of the surrounding tissues, which should be preserved.

If the osteoclast is located on a flat surface, the localized bone resorption results in a concavity or *resorption lacuna* (Howship's lacuna). At the end of the resorption period a bone surface may have many of these concavities.

Arrest Lines and Reversal Lines

The study of a histologic section of bone can reveal much of the history of this tissue. A layer of osteoblasts involved in bone deposition occasionally takes a rest stop before continuing with further bone deposition. In the bone tissue such a rest stop shows up as a deeply staining *arrest line*. Arrest lines are relatively smooth. They consist of intercellular substance with a slightly different proportion of collagen and ground substance from that present in the rest of the tissue. Because of this, arrest lines stain differently (they are more acid) and remain visible in the bone tissue formed before and after the rest stop (Fig. 5–13, *A*).

Reversal lines are lines that stain much the same as arrest lines, but reversal lines are scalloped, not smooth. They represent the terminal location of a series of resorption lacunae. Following the termination of the resorption process, new osteoblasts differentiated and deposited bone tissue. Thus, the resorption cavities were filled with new bone, and the bone surface was gradually smoothed in the process (Fig. 5–13, *B*).

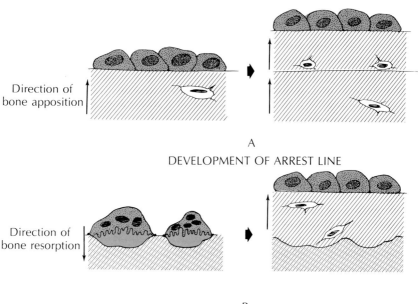

A

DEVELOPMENT OF ARREST LINE

B

DEVELOPMENT OF REVERSAL LINE

Fig. 5–13. *A, An arrest line is formed in bone when the process of bone deposition, by a layer of osteoblasts, is temporarily halted and subsequently resumed. The small arrows indicate the direction in which the bone surface moves. B, A reversal line is formed in bone when the process of bone resorption, by a layer of osteoclasts, is halted and followed by the deposition of a new layer of bone by osteoblasts. The small arrows indicate the opposite directions, in which the bone surface moves during the resorption and the apposition of bone. Since a bone surface, which undergoes bone deposition, is smooth, an arrest line is smooth. Since resorption creates resorption lacunae on a bone surface, a reversal line, reflecting the final resorption surface, is scalloped.*

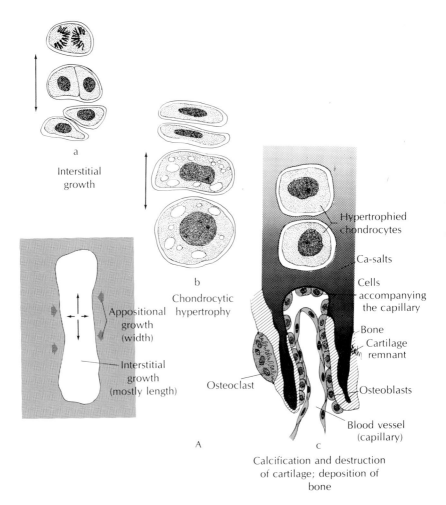

Fig. 5–14. **A,** *In a cartilaginously preformed model of a long bone most appositional growth results in an increase in width of the model, while interstitial growth is largely responsible for the increase in length. In a we show diagrammatically how, during this interstitial growth, the cells stack vertically into a column after mitosis. The next event, illustrated in b, hypertrophy of the chondrocytes, also leads to an increase in the vertical dimensions of the cartilage mass. In the final stages of chondrocytic hypertrophy, the cartilage matrix, between the columns of hypertrophied chondrocytes, is calcified. Once the matrix is calcified, the cartilage can be resorbed and replaced by bone. As illustrated in c, small blood vessels grow toward this calcified cartilage. Some mesenchymal cells, which accompany them, break down most of the cartilage. Other cells come along with the blood vessels, differentiate into osteoblasts and begin to deposit bone on the cartilage remnants. This new bone is not long lived. Remodeling (by osteoclasts) soon follows, removing most of the young bone and leaving behind a marrow cavity. As is stated in the text, b and c must occur before endochondral ossification can take place. Although a usually precedes b and c, it is not a necessary condition for endochondral ossification.*

Formation of
primary ossi-
fication
center

Formation of
secondary
ossification
centers.

Mature bone

B

B, *Three stages in the ossification of a long bone in the limb are illustrated.* Formation of a primary ossification center: *The earliest destruction of cartilage and replacement by bone occur in the middle of the shaft of a long bone model. The processes then continue, in 2 opposite directions, toward the ends of the model. Notice that most of the cartilage is not replaced by bone and that a large central marrow cavity remains.* Formation of secondary ossification centers: *In the cartilage masses at the ends of the long bone model, smaller, separate ossification centers are established. Endochondral ossification spreads in these areas from the center towards the periphery. Note that 2 narrow plates of cartilage remain between the primary and secondary ossification centers. These are the growth plates of the long bone. They are responsible for the further (interstitial) growth in length of the bone and will remain in existence until skeletal maturity is reached and growth ceases. In these growth plates endochondral ossification, as illustrated in Fig. 5–14 A, continues. At puberty the growth plates disappear. The long bone now consists entirely of bone, with a central marrow cavity. Some spongy bone is found near the ends, but most of the shaft consists of compact lamellar bone, with many osteons. The 2 joint surfaces at the ends remain covered with hyaline cartilage throughout the individual's life.*

Endochondral Ossification

In areas where there is an early need for skeletal support, during prenatal development, some bones are preformed as cartilaginous models. The advantage of such cartilage models is that they provide early, resilient support for the developing body and, at the same time, serve as important sites of growth. Remember that bone can only grow by apposition, whereas cartilage grows both apposition-ally *and* interstitially.

Bone tissue gradually *replaces* the cartilage models. This is done by breakdown of the cartilage tissue, in localized areas, and deposition of bone tissue on the cartilage remnants. The cartilage must undergo 2 important changes before it can be broken down and replaced by bone: chondrocytic hypertrophy and cartilage matrix calcification.

In *chondrocytic hypertrophy* the individual chondrocytes increase in size. These cells become much larger and vacuolated, and then degenerate.

In *cartilage matrix calcification* the degenerating chondrocytes deposit hydroxyapatite salts in the cartilage matrix.

The process of endochondral ossification in the skull is rather complex, and so we will demonstrate its principles on one of the long limb bones, which also form by endochondral ossification (Fig. 5–14).

Chondrocytic hypertrophy and cartilage calcification occur first in the middle and then slowly spread toward the 2 ends of the long bone model. Simultaneously, a collar of bone is deposited by osteoblasts on the outside surface of the cartilage, at the level of the earliest cartilage changes. This bone collar expands toward the 2 ends of the model at approximately the same rate at which the cartilage changes spread inside the model. The bone collar serves as an external scaffold, taking over the support function of the changed cartilage tissue, which will be removed.

A blood vessel, accompanied by differentiating osteoblasts and osteoclasts, invades the cartilage model and begins its destruction and replacement. The calcified cartilage with the hypertrophic chondrocytes is invaded by numerous branches of this blood vessel. The osteoclasts remove much of the calcified intercellular substance. On some of the cartilage remnants the osteoblasts begin to deposit bone tissue. While the already changed cartilage is thus broken down and replaced by the first bone trabeculae, the processes of chondrocytic hypertrophy and cartilage calcification spread further in opposite directions, toward the 2 ends of the cartilage model.

If no further growth activity would take place in the remainder of the cartilage model, the process of its replacement would be finished rapidly. However, before the chondrocytes hypertrophy and participate in the calcification of the intercellular substance, they usually undergo several mitoses, thus enlarging the cartilage model interstitially.

In the long bones all growth in length is due to the interstitial growth of the cartilage, before it is replaced by bone. Once bone tissue has replaced the cartilage, only appositional growth is possible, leading largely to an increase in the width of these bones. No bone forms on the joint surfaces at the ends of the bones. These remain covered with hyaline cartilage, which is able to resist the compressive loading placed on the joint surfaces in function. Once all the cartilage of the original model is removed (with the exception of the cartilage on the joint surfaces), the growth in length of the long bone stops. Any further bone formation can only produce a wider bone with greater density, but not a longer bone.

Frequently, more than one site of bone formation is found in the cartilage model of a long bone. Such *ossification centers* spread individually, so that soon only narrow strips of cartilage, *growth plates,* remain. Usually, 2 growth plates are found in the long bones of growing individuals. When skeletal maturity is reached, generally in the teenage years, the chondrocytes in the growth plates stop undergoing mitoses. The remaining cells hypertrophy, the cartilage is calcified, and then the whole growth plate is broken down and replaced with bone.

Once endochondral ossification is completed and the growing cartilages are resorbed, the individual bone has attained its final length. However, if a growth cartilage is destroyed *before* it has stopped growing, for instance, as the result of an accident or a bad infection, further growth in length of the bone is halted, and it will be abnormally short for the rest of the individual's life. A well-known example of what can happen to the growth of long bones, when the cartilage stops growing before sexual maturity is reached, is poliomyelitis, affecting a growing person.

JOINTS

Joints are the structures between 2 adjacent bones. The following joints are found in the skull (Fig. 5–15): sutures, synchondroses, and the temporomandibular joint.

SUTURES. Sutures are dense, fibrous connections between adjacent *intramembranously* formed bones. Some minor movements between these bones are made possible by the sutures. Sutures have several functions:

1. They allow passage through the narrow birth canal by letting adjacent bones of the skull overlap, thus temporarily reducing the size of the skull.

2. They serve as shock breakers. If sutures were not present, the skull would more easily fracture on impact.

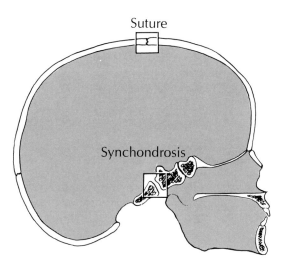

Fig. 5–15. *Diagram, showing locations of a suture and a synchondrosis in a child's skull. A third type of joint, the temporomandibular joint, is found between the lower jaw and the rest of the skull, just in front of the ear. There are several sutures in the skull, many of which remain visible throughout life. During fetal life, there are also several synchondroses in the endochondrally ossifying skull base. Only one of these, however, persists after birth until skeletal maturity is reached. This synchondrosis, the spheno-occipital synchondrosis, is illustrated in this figure.*

Fig. 5–16. *Suture in a histologic section through the midline of the hard palate in a young primate. The 2 bone edges are visible with several distinct layers of intervening soft tissues; cellular layer, mostly osteoblasts (C), and fibrous layer (F) of the periosteum of one bone edge (P1) and cellular and fibrous layers of the periosteum (P2) covering the second bone edge form a sandwich arrangement with a richly vascularized middle layer. In this last layer collagen fibers run obliquely between the 2 periostea (P1 and P2). A reversal line (R) and several arrest lines (A) are visible in the bones themselves, attesting to a certain amount of bone remodeling in the suture. Original magnification × 100.*

98

3. They serve as sites of appositional bone growth during the period of growth. This results in an increase in the size of the individual bones and thus in an increase in overall skull size.

Histologically, a suture is composed of the meeting edges of the adjacent bones, their periosteal coverings and an intermediate connective tissue layer.

The bone edges may be smooth or irregular, straight or beveled. Each bone is covered with a layer of periosteum, composed of an inner layer of osteoblasts and occasionally osteoclasts, next to the bone surface, and an outer fibrous layer. The osteoblasts are capable of increasing the dimensions of the bone by appositional growth. If the dimensions of the individual bones increase, the skull as a whole increases in size. Between the 2 opposing fibrous layers of periosteum a middle layer is present. This layer consists of dense connective tissue, with many collagen fibers running from one fibrous layer to the other. The middle layer also contains the blood supply for the periosteal osteoblasts (Fig. 5–16).

SYNCHONDROSES. A synchondrosis is a cartilaginous joint between 2 adjacent endochondrally formed bones of the skull. This joint allows little movement between the bones, as well as further endochondral ossification at the facing ends of the 2 adjacent bones. This increases the size of these bones.

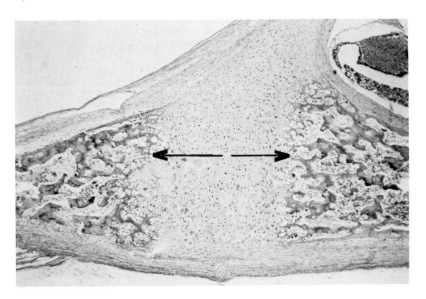

Fig. 5–17. Midline section through the spheno-occipital synchondrosis in the skull base of a newborn primate. The surface facing the brain is at the top, while the surface facing the pharynx is at the bottom. The cartilaginous synchondrosis undergoes the processes of endochondral ossification at both ends (arrows), somewhat resembling a bipolar growth plate. Original magnification × 12.5.

Synchondroses are found in the skull base of a growing individual and the interstitial cartilage growth in these structures enlarges the skull base in a direction from front to back. One synchondrosis, the spheno-occipital synchondrosis (located between sphenoid and occipital bones), continues to undergo endochondral ossification until skeletal maturity at about 16 years of age. At that time it generally disappears. The structure of a synchondrosis resembles 2 growth plates mounted "back to back." We call this structure bipolar, which means that endochondral ossification takes place at both ends of a synchondrosis, leading to an increase in the length of the bones of the cranial base and of the cranial base itself (Fig. 5–17).

   TEMPOROMANDIBULAR JOINT. The joint between the mandible and the rest of the skull, the temporomandibular joint, is the only joint in the skull with joint cavities, making this a freely moveable joint. The joint is between the endochondrally formed part of the mandible, the *condylar head* (the rest of the mandible is formed by intramembranous ossification), and the intramembranously formed articular tubercle on the zygomatic process of the temporal bone. The structure of the joint is shown in Figure 5–18. Since both the mandibular condyle and the articular tubercle have convex surfaces, a bi-concave disc of dense collagenous connective tissue intervenes between the 2 surfaces, to make them compatible for joint motion.

   The articular surfaces of the temporomandibular joint are somewhat unlike the joint surfaces of most other joints in the body in that they are covered with dense fibrous, collagenous tissue (later in life they are covered with fibrocartilage) rather than with hyaline cartilage.

   The increase in height of the ramus of the mandible is made possible by the endochondral ossification process taking place in the mandibular condyle. In growing individuals the condyle consists of a mass of hyaline cartilage, in which the chondrocytes are undergoing

Fig. 5–18. A, *Histologic section through the temporomandibular joint of a young primate. AT = articular tubercle; D = articular disc; C = mandibular condylar head. The articular disc and the covering layers of the articular tubercle and mandibular condylar head consist of dense collagenous, fibrous connective tissue. Between the bone and the fibrous layer of the articular tubercle a darkly staining layer of calcified cartilage is present. In the mandibular condylar head endochondral ossification of the hyaline cartilage layer is taking place, allowing for vertical growth of that part of the lower jaw. There is little interstitial growth in this cartilage. Most growth is the result of the appositional activities of the chondroblasts, located underneath the fibrous layer* (arrow). *When skeletal maturity is reached, most cartilage will be replaced by bone in the condylar head, which will resemble histologically the articular tubercle. Original magnification × 10. B, The temporomandibular joint of a young adult man, seen in histologic section. AT = articular tubercle; D = articular disc; C = mandibular condylar head. Some fibers of the lateral pterygoid muscle are visible, inserting into the periosteum of the neck of the condyle* (arrow). *The upper and the lower joint cavities appear as light spaces. In the back, part of a section through the joint capsule is seen (at the right side). Original magnification × 2 (Courtesy the late Dr. E. Applebaum.)*

hypertrophy and the cartilage matrix becomes calcified. Typical endochondral ossification is occurring, but at a slow pace. Little interstitial growth is taking place in this cartilage. We see mostly *appositional* growth here, with a layer of chondroblasts located underneath the fibrous articular surface layer. The process of endochondral ossification is completed between the ages of 18 and 30 years. At that time all hyaline cartilage underneath the fibrous layer is calcified and/or replaced by bone tissue.

The *articular tubercle* is also covered with a fibrous layer. This may become fibrocartilage in the deeper areas of this layer, which covers the bone of the tubercle directly.

Surrounding the temporomandibular joint components is an *articular capsule,* consisting of an outer layer of dense fibrous connective tissue and an inner layer of loose connective tissue, with a rich network of blood vessels. The innermost lining or *synovial lining* of this capsule, which faces directly the joint cavities (upper and lower, separated from each other by the *articular disc*), consists of a layer of fibroblasts. These cells produce carbohydrate-rich substances, which are added to the fluid that has filtered out of the blood vessels. This filtered fluid with the carbohydrate-rich substances is the *synovia,* the lubricant of the joint cavities.

On the outer surface of the joint capsule, at the level of the disc, and on the neck of the mandibular condyle, 2 parts of the lateral pterygoid muscle attach. This muscle moves both disc and condyle forward during mouth opening and is one of the 4 *masticatory* muscles.

SELECTED READING LIST

Bloom, W., and Bloom, M.A.: Calcification and ossification. Calcification of developing bones in embryonic and newborn rats. Anat. Rec., 78:497, 1940.

Durkin, J., Heeley, J., and Irving, J.T.: The cartilage of the mandibular condyle. Oral Sciences Rev., 2:29, 1973.

Enlow, D.H.: The Human Face. An Account of the Postnatal Growth and Development of the Craniofacial Skeleton. New York, Harper & Row, 1968.

Gardner, E.: Osteogenesis in the human embryo and fetus. In The Biochemistry and Physiology of Bone. Volume III. Development and Growth. 2nd Ed. Edited by G.H. Bourne, New York, Academic Press, 1971.

Hall, B.K.: Cellular differentiation in skeletal tissues. Biol. Rev., 45:455, 1970.

———: The origin and fate of osteoclasts. Anat. Rec., 183:1, 1975.

Hancox, N.M.: Biology of Bone. London, Cambridge University Press, 1972.

Lacroix, P.: The internal remodeling of bones. In The Biochemistry and Physiology of Bone. Volume III. Development and Growth. 2nd Ed. Edited by G.H. Bourne. New York, Academic Press, 1971.

Lentz, T.: Cell Fine Structure. An Atlas of Drawings of Whole Cell Structure. Philadelphia, W.B. Saunders Co., 1971.

Sissons, H.A.: The growth of bone. In The Biochemistry and Physiology of Bone. Volume III. Development and Growth. 2nd Ed. Edited by G. H. Bourne. New York, Academic Press, 1971.

Sperber, G.H.: Craniofacial Embryology. 2nd Ed. Dental Practitioner Handbook #15. Bristol, John Wright and Sons, 1976.

Vaughan, J.: The Physiology of Bone. 2nd Ed. Oxford, Clarendon Press, 1975.

Chapter 6

MUSCLE AND NERVE TISSUE; BLOOD VESSELS AND BLOOD; LYMPHATICS

During inspection of the oral cavity, you may observe that some parts, such as the lips and cheeks, tongue and soft palate, can be moved at will. These parts contain a central core of *muscle tissue,* a tissue specialized in contractions, which is responsible for the observed movements.

In this chapter we will have a closer look at the constituents of muscle tissue and their relationship to the other structures of the oral cavity. In addition, we will describe components of 2 other systems essential to the function and maintenance of tissues around the oral cavity: the *vascular* system and the *nervous* system. The chapter will end with a brief description of lymph vessels and lymphatic tissue, as they relate to the orofacial region.

MUSCLE TISSUE

Muscle tissue consists predominantly of *cells* that have differentiated from embryonic mesenchymal cells to become highly specialized in *contracting* or shortening. This specialization, compared with specialization in other cell types, involves the production of considerable amounts of *intracellular,* contractile protein filaments. These protein filaments largely determine the appearance of the muscle cells, because of their abundance and their organization inside the muscle cells and also because of their staining properties.

The contraction of the individual muscle cells would have little effect on the tissues to be moved as the result of the muscle contraction if these muscle cells were not organized, packed together, and tied to each other and the surrounding tissues in a specific manner. Muscle tissue proper consists of *specialized muscle cells* that are bound together functionally by a *connective tissue framework.* This same connective tissue also carries the rich blood vessel and nerve supplies needed for the function of the muscle.

There are 3 *types* of muscle tissue: skeletal (striated) muscle tissue, smooth muscle tissue, and heart muscle tissue.

SKELETAL (STRIATED) MUSCLE TISSUE. In skeletal muscles, contractions are generally under our own control and are therefore called *voluntary.* By and large, these contractions are rapid, short in duration and powerful (although these characteristics may show some variation, depending on the type of muscle and the nature of the work it has to perform).

Skeletal muscle contractions are initiated by stimuli of motor nerves (this chapter). These muscles are found wherever skeletal elements are to be moved, relative to each other (example: masticatory muscles between the mandible and the rest of the skull); where the skin has to be moved relative to underlying skeletal elements (example: muscles of facial expression, between facial bones and facial skin); and where a muscular organ (the tongue) has to be moved relative to the lower jaw (muscles running from several points of the skull into the tongue) or has to change its own shape (muscles running inside the tongue only).

SMOOTH MUSCLE TISSUE. In smooth muscle tissue, the contractions generally do not require our conscious control, although they may be brought under our control with a good deal of practice. These *involuntary* muscle contractions are under the control of our autonomic nervous system. They are slow, but may be maintained over long periods of time without the use of much energy. This is quite in contrast with contractions of skeletal muscles, which require a great deal of energy and rapidly exhaust the muscles.

Structures in which smooth muscle tissue is found include the walls of the stomach, intestines, urinary bladder, uterus and *arteries.*

HEART MUSCLE TISSUE. This type of muscle tissue has characteristics of both skeletal and smooth muscle tissue. It is an *involuntary* muscle, capable of fast, powerful contractions. This type of muscle will not be discussed further here, since it is beyond the scope of this text.

Organization of Skeletal Muscle Tissue

The organization of a skeletal muscle is best illustrated by the structure of a cut of meat (most meat that we eat consists of skeletal muscle). Meat, or skeletal muscle tissue, is usually not homogeneous, but may be separated into distinct parts or *bundles.* The separation takes place along connective tissue sheaths, which cover and surround the muscle bundles (as well as the individual muscle fibers). Connective tissue also ties the muscle bundles to each other and to the dense, highly organized connective tissue sheath, which surrounds the entire muscle (Fig. 6–1).

If you take part of a muscle bundle and gently tease it with a fine

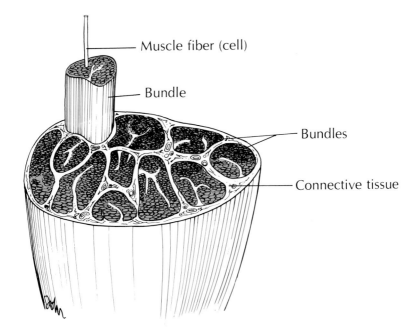

Muscle fiber (cell)

Bundle

Bundles

Connective tissue

Fig. 6–1. Diagram of the structure of a small skeletal muscle. The entire muscle is surrounded by a thick connective tissue sheath (epimysium). Within the muscle several smaller bundles of muscle fibers are present, each of which is surrounded by a thin connective tissue sheath (perimysium). The individual muscle fibers, of which a fiber bundle is composed, each have their own delicate connective tissue sheaths (endomysium).

needle, you will be able to separate it into fine strands, which are called *muscle fibers.* (Note: These muscle *fibers* are in fact *muscle cells* and are *not* comparable to the intercellular fibers of connective tissues.)

The reason skeletal muscle cells are visible with the unaided eye is their large size. Striated muscle cells may be 30 to 100 μm thick and up to 300 mm long. These unusual cell dimensions are produced during the prenatal development of striated muscle. The large cells actually are produced as the result of *fusion* of many differentiating mesenchymal cells. This fusion produces one giant cell, with many oval-shaped nuclei (Fig. 6–2).

Skeletal, or striated, muscle cells are shaped like elongated cylinders, with rounded ends. Their cytoplasm contains large amounts of tightly packed bundles of contractile protein-filaments, seemingly pushing the nuclei and other organelles, such as the mitochondria, to the sides of the cell.

The bundles of contractile protein-filaments, located inside the cell, are about 1 μm thick and are therefore visible with the light

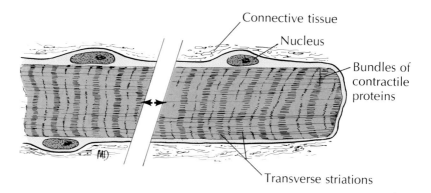

Fig. 6–2. *Simplified diagram of a striated muscle fiber (cell). This big cell has blunt, rounded ends and many oval nuclei, all peripherally located within a thin band of cytoplasm. Most of the cell's volume is occupied by bundles of contractile protein filaments with cross-striations. A delicate connective tissue sheath, predominantly consisting of reticulin fibers, surrounds the entire cell. The double-headed arrow indicates that this cell type is far too long to be shown in its entirety in this diagram.*

microscope. They have cross striations along their length. Many of these bundles neatly line up inside the muscle cell, making it appear as if the cell itself is striated. These cross striations are responsible for the name *striated muscle,* which is frequently used for skeletal muscle. In the section on muscle contractions, we will briefly discuss the structural basis for these striations.

The following is a *summary* of the organization of a skeletal muscle from the cellular level to the anatomically identifiable muscle (Fig. 6–1).

1. Individual *muscle cells* (fibers) are surrounded by a delicate connective tissue sheath, consisting predominantly of reticulin fibers. This sheath fits around an individual muscle cell like a "body stocking."

2. A group of cells, with their reticular sheaths, is packed together in a *bundle,* surrounded by a layer of connective tissue consisting predominantly of collagen fibers.

3. Several bundles together form a *muscle,* which is surrounded by a layer of dense connective tissue.

The *connective tissue frame* around cells, bundles and whole mass of a skeletal muscle performs important functions: biomechanical support functions and nutritional functions.

Biomechanical Support Functions

1. The connective tissue frame supports the individual muscle cells and holds them together in a particular orientation and shape.

2. Because of their intimate contacts with all individual muscle cells, the connective tissue elements *transmit* the *contractions* of these cells to the connective tissue at the points of attachment of the muscle.

3. The connective tissue frame of the muscle *binds* the muscle to its points of attachment, either *directly,* by forming numerous short fibers, which run into periosteum, perichondrium, lamina propria of the oral mucosa, or dermis of the skin; or *indirectly,* by attaching the muscle mass to a highly oriented rope (tendon) or sheet (aponeurosis) of collagenous connective tissue, which in turn inserts into a skeletal element (see skeletal muscle attachments, below).

Nutritional Functions

The connective tissue elements between muscle bundles contain blood vessels and nerves, both of which branch inside this connective tissue into progressively finer branches. A rich network is formed of fine blood vessels inside the connective tissue elements around the individual muscle cells, and each cell is innervated by one nerve fiber.

The rich vascularization is responsible in part for the red color of muscle tissue. The contents of the muscle cells themselves further contribute to this color.

Skeletal Muscle Attachments

Skeletal muscle attachments are formed by elements of its connective tissue frame. The precise nature of an attachment depends on the site and the function of the muscle. For example, the muscle tissue, which by its contraction changes the *shape* of the *tongue,* is attached on both sides to the lamina propria of the oral mucosa of the tongue. In contrast to this, the muscles which, by their contraction, *move* the *tongue* relative to the skeletal elements are attached on one end only to the oral mucosa of the tongue and on the other end to the skeletal element in question. The muscles of *facial expression* either attach with both ends into the dermis of the skin or, more frequently, attach with one end to the skin and with the other end to the skeleton. Certain muscles in the *lips* attach with one end into the skin and with the other into the oral mucosa. Their contractions change the thickness and shape of the lips. *Masticatory* muscles, which move the lower jaw complex relative to the rest of the skull, attach with both ends to skeletal elements.

In many instances, the connective tissue elements, which surround and support the muscle components, run directly into the *periosteum* when the attachment is to bone, into the *perichondrium* when the attachment is to cartilage, into the *dermis* when the attachments is to skin, or into the *lamina propria* when the attachment is to oral mucosa. The collagen fibers of the connective tissue frame mesh with the meshwork of collagen fibers in any of these structures, thus fastening the muscle securely to them.

Occasionally, an intermediate structure, a *tendon,* may be involved in the muscle attachment. This may be a heavy, rope-like structure, or a sheet-like tendon, sometimes called *aponeurosis.* If a tendon is present, the connective tissue elements of the muscle mesh with the collagen fibers of the tendon. The tendon itself consists of dense connective tissue, with highly oriented and compacted collagen fibers. This structure may insert into periosteum or perichondrium, but in some locations it runs directly into the bone tissue. The tendon fibers, which are embedded in the bone, become calcified (hydroxyapatite is deposited in them) to a large extent.

Because of the dense organization of a tendon, its fibroblasts are compressed between the thick cords of collagen fibers. These are *not* actively synthesizing cells, and the turnover time of tendon components is long.

The vascular supply of a tendon is minimal, reflecting this tissue's low metabolic activity. Blood vessels tend to run inside narrow strands of loose connective tissue, interposed between the thick collagen fibers. We will see later a similar arrangement in the principal fiber bundles of the periodontal ligament. Because of its minimal blood supply and its low metabolic activity, a ruptured tendon does not heal readily.

Organization of Smooth Muscle Tissue

In the orofacial area, smooth muscle cells are found in the wall of the trachea and in the walls of blood vessels, mostly arteries and arterioles. Smooth muscle cells are somewhat longer than most other cells in the body, but they are by no means as long as the striated muscle cells. Their lengths are between 15 and 500 μm and their diameters between 5 and 10 μm. Whereas striated muscle cells are large conglomerates, formed prenatally by fusion of many differentiating mesenchymal cells, the smooth muscle cells are formed prenatally by *single,* differentiating, mesenchymal cells.

Smooth muscle cells are elongated and spindle-shaped, with one long, sausage-shaped nucleus. This nucleus is located centrally in the cell. While contractile protein-filaments, somewhat similar in nature to those in striated muscle cells, are present in substantial amounts in the smooth muscle cytoplasm, they are far less strictly organized than in striated muscle cells and they are not visible in the light microscope (Fig. 6–3).

Each striated muscle cell is individually innervated, but only a few smooth muscle cells are innervated. Nevertheless, smooth

Connective tissue sheath

Fig. 6–3.   A simplified diagram of a smooth muscle cell. This long, spindle-shaped cell has a single, sausage-shaped nucleus, which is located centrally. The protein filaments in the cytoplasm of these cells are not as strictly organized as the filaments in striated muscle cells, and they are not visible by light microscopy. A delicate "stocking" of reticulin fibers surrounds the cell.

muscle cells can contract in an organized and coordinated fashion. This is because once the impulse for contraction is received by the few innervated cells, this impulse is immediately communicated to the non-innervated cells via the low-resistance *gap junctions,* by which the smooth muscle cells are functionally coupled.

Each individual smooth muscle cell is surrounded by its connective tissue "body-stocking," consisting mainly of reticulin fibers, except in the areas of the gap junctions.

As in striated muscle, a connective tissue frame with both biomechanical and nutritional functions is associated with an organized group of smooth muscle cells. Since smooth muscle cells tend to be located in the walls of hollow structures, such as blood vessels, the mechanical functions of the connective tissue consist largely of the *transmission* of muscle contraction, which decreases the size or diameter of the hollow structure, and the provision of *mechanical support* for the muscle cells and the wall of the hollow structure itself.

Mechanism of Muscle Contraction

Although the principles of muscle contraction appear to be comparable in both smooth and striated muscle cells, most investigations on muscle contraction have been performed on striated muscle cells. Their high degree of organization enables us to give a simple account of muscle contraction, without going into the intricate physiology of the contraction process, for which the interested reader is referred to more extensive texts on this particular subject.

As may be seen in Figure 6–4, the cytoplasm of a striated muscle cell contains many *bundles* of contractile protein-filaments. The organization of these protein-filaments within the bundles is shown.

The bundles of contractile protein-filaments in a striated muscle cell are usually called *myofibrils.* Each myofibril, in turn, consists of regularly arranged protein-filaments, *actin* and *myosin* filaments. In regularly stained histologic sections, the darker striations are pro-

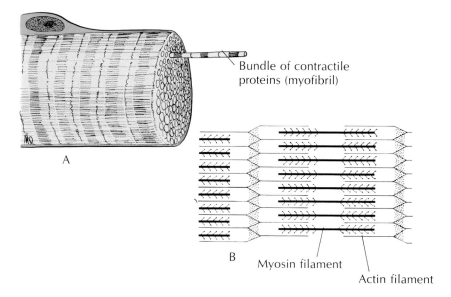

Bundle of contractile proteins (myofibril)

A

B   Myosin filament

Actin filament

Fig. 6–4. From the cut end of a striated muscle cell, shown in this diagram, one bundle of contractile proteins (a myofibril) protrudes, A, A small segment of this myofibril is enlarged, B, to show the arrangement of the protein filaments (actin and myosin filaments), that are responsible for the striations and for the contraction mechanism. The stippled, vertical bands are the Z-lines. Actin filaments are attached back to back to the Z-lines. The heavier myosin filaments alternate with the actin filaments. The segment between 2 Z-lines is a sarcomere, the unit of contraction of a striated muscle cell.

duced by the presence of the myosin filaments, while the lighter areas contain only actin filaments. The actin filaments are attached "back-to-back" to a "backbone" or *Z-line*. That section of a myofibril that is located between 2 Z-lines is the contractile unit or *sarcomere* of the myofibril. Each sarcomere is composed of one dark striation and 2 half light striations.

During muscle contraction, the actin and myosin filaments slide past each other, thereby shortening the lengths of the individual

Fig. 6–5. Two diagrams of a sarcomere, the unit of contraction of a striated muscle cell, located between 2 Z-lines (dark vertical bands). During contraction, the actin filaments slide past the myosin filaments toward each other, bringing the 2 Z-lines closer together and thus decreasing the length of the sarcomere (arrows). If this occurs simultaneously in all sarcomeres along the length of a muscle fiber, this fiber shortens considerably.

Table 6–1.   Nomenclature of Striated Muscle Tissue

Intracellular structures

Myofibrils	Bundles of contractile protein-filaments found in the muscle fibers.
Myofilaments	Contractile protein-filaments, composed of the contractile proteins actin and myosin.
Sarcomere	The contractile unit of a myofibril.
Sarcolemma	The outer membrane of a muscle fiber, consisting of the lipoprotein membrane of the cell, plus a basal lamina
Sarcoplasm	The cytoplasm of the muscle cell.
Sarcoplasmic reticulum	A modified type of agranular endoplasmic reticulum, composed of tubules and cisternae; it is found in the sarcoplasm and forms a canalicular arrangement around each myofibril.
Transverse tubules (T-tubules)	A narrow transverse tubule that extends inward from the sarcolemma. Two cisternae of the sarcoplasmic reticulum are found on either side of the T-tubule. This arrangement is referred to as the *triad* of the reticulum. In human skeletal muscle there are two triads per sarcomere. The T-tubules play a vital role in facilitating skeletal muscle contraction. When a nerve impulse is propagated along a nerve fiber, in the area where the motor-endplate meets the muscle, the sarcolemma lining the synaptic trough becomes permeable to ions. The increase in flow of the ions generates an action potential, and a wave of depolarization spreads over the entire muscle fiber and into its interior via the T-tubule system, thus causing the muscle to contract.

Connective tissue frame structures

Epimysium	The thick, highly organized, connective tissue layer that encloses the muscle as a whole. Gross anatomically known as *fascia*.
Perimysium	The connective tissue layer that envelops a *bundle* of muscle fibers.
Endomysium	The connective tissue that extends from the perimysium into the muscle bundle. This connective tissue branches into progressively finer branches, until each individual muscle fiber or cell is surrounded by a delicate sheath (the "body stocking").

sarcomeres in a fashion known as the sliding mechanism. The shortening of the individual sarcomeres leads to the shortening of the total length of the muscle cell, which is somewhat more than the sum of all sarcomeres (Fig. 6–5).

NERVE TISSUE

The nervous system, composed of nerve tissue, might be compared with a large central computer (*central nervous system:* brain

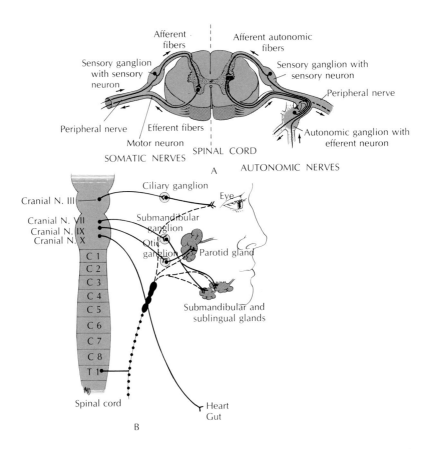

Fig. 6–6. A, Some pathways of the peripheral nervous system, leading into and out of a section of spinal cord, are shown in this diagram. The spinal cord is seen from the front. For clarity, pathways of autonomic nerves are illustrated on the right side, while pathways of somatic nerves are shown on the left side. It should be understood that both types of nerves are found on both sides. Input signals (afferent) reach the sensory neurons in the peripherally located sensory ganglia. These signals may then be transmitted further centrally, where the motor neurons and autonomic neurons are located. From these neurons, output signals (efferent) may leave the central nervous system for an appropriate peripheral response. Notice that the autonomic output signals use 2 autonomic neurons (one whose cell body is located in the spinal cord and one whose cell body is located in a peripheral autonomic ganglion). The somatic output signals use only one neuron, the cell body of which is located in the spinal cord, while the input signals similarly use only one neuron, the cell body of which is located in a peripheral sensory ganglion. B, The autonomic pathways for the head and neck region are shown in this diagram. The sympathetic outflow comes from the thoracic level of the spinal cord (dotted line from T1). The second group of neuronal cell bodies is located in the superior cervical ganglion (black). From there all sympathetic output signals travel further along nerve fibers, associated with blood vessels (broken lines). The parasympathetic neurons are located in the brain. Parasympathetic output signals travel in nerve fibers associated with 4 cranial nerves. A second group of neuronal cell bodies is located in 4 parasympathetic ganglia. From those, the parasympathetic output signals travel further toward the viscera (especially salivary glands) that are innervated by them (solid lines). For clarity, the fourth parasympathetic ganglion in this area, the pterygopalatine ganglion, has been omitted from this diagram. Parasympathetic signals from this ganglion travel to all parts of face and pharynx.

and spinal cord) with numerous input and output channels (*peripheral nervous system:* nerves and small aggregates of nerve cells [ganglia]).

In Figure 6–6 some pathways of the nervous system are shown. There are nerves that transmit impulses from the periphery to the central nervous system (example: sensation in the skin is transmitted this way via *afferent nerves;* this is *sensory input*). Other nerves transmit impulses or commands from the central nervous system to the periphery. (Example: the impulse for contraction of a skeletal muscle is transmitted this way, via *efferent nerves;* this is somatic, motor output. Another example: the impulse for secretion in a salivary gland is transmitted this way: via efferent nerves; this is *autonomic,* secretomotor output.) In the central nervous system, the input is sorted out and processed. When necessary the information is converted into appropriate output signals.

Within the nervous system, we distinguish 2 principal types of *cells:*

1. Nerve cells or *neurons:* involved in impulse transmission. The cell bodies of these cells are located in the central nervous system or in the peripheral nervous system, in the ganglia. The long processes of these cells are located in the peripheral nerves.

2. Supporting cells: *glia cells* in the central nervous system; *Schwann cells* in the peripheral nerves; and *satellite cells* in the ganglia. These cells are involved in support and service functions of the nervous system.

NEURONS. Neurons are cells that are specialized in the conduction of impulses (an electric current flow) along their cell membranes. The differentiated neuron is no longer capable of mitoses. A neuron generally consists of a relatively large cell body (4 to 135 μm) and one, two or more cell processes, which may be of variable lengths. The number and the lengths of these processes depend on the location of the neuron within the communication system.

1. The neurons of the *central nervous system* and in the *autonomic ganglia* have several cell processes *(multipolar neurons).* Usually one of these, the *axon,* is considerably longer than the others *(dendrites).* Dendrites generally receive and conduct impulses *toward* the neuronal *cell body.* The axon conducts impulses *away* from the cell body (Fig. 6–7).

Numerous cell contacts *(synapses)* exist between the neurons in the central nervous system, resulting in a very complex circuitry. Within the central nervous system, groups of neurons, *centers,* subserve specific functions in processing sensory information and control of motor output. Many of these cells do not have cell processes beyond the central nervous system.

2. Neurons in *sensory ganglia* have one single process that later bifurcates (T-shape). These are called *pseudo-unipolar neurons* (Fig. 6–7).

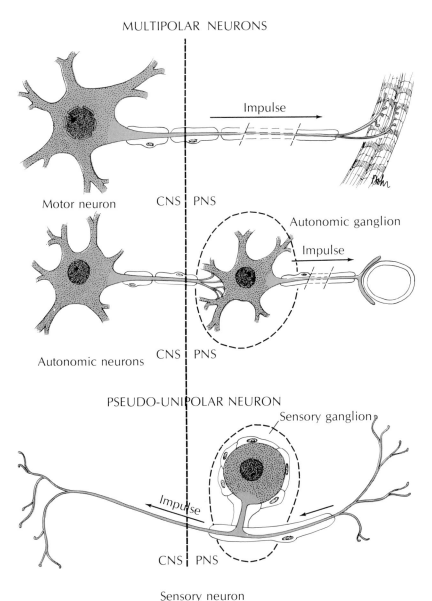

MULTIPOLAR NEURONS

Impulse

Motor neuron

CNS | PNS

Autonomic ganglion

Impulse

Autonomic neurons

CNS | PNS

PSEUDO-UNIPOLAR NEURON

Sensory ganglion

Impulse

CNS | PNS

Sensory neuron

Fig. 6–7. Diagrammatic representation of 3 multipolar neurons and one pseudo-unipolar neuron. The vertical broken line in all diagrams represents the border between central nervous system (CNS) and peripheral nervous system (PNS). The arrows indicate the direction in which the signal impulses move. One of the cell processes of a multipolar motor neuron, whose cell body is located in the CNS, is a very long axon, innervating a skeletal muscle. Some light, supporting cells (Schwann cells) are illustrated along the length of the axon. Of the 2 autonomic multipolar neurons, one is located in the CNS. Its axon communicates with a second multipolar neuron in an autonomic ganglion. From this cell a second axon runs toward the structure to be innervated (a blood vessel in this case). Supporting cells are illustrated around the axons. A neuron in a sensory ganglion is pseudo-unipolar. One cell process leaves the cell body, but it divides almost immediately into 2 long branches: one running toward the CNS and one running toward the periphery of the body (skin, oral mucosa). The impulse travels in the direction of the arrows from periphery to CNS.

The maintenance of the long cell processes of a neuron (especially a motor neuron, whose cell body lies in the central nervous system, while its cell process, the axon, ends in a skeletal muscle) is demanding and therefore the cell body is actively engaged in protein synthesis. A constant flow of proteins takes place in the axon from the cell body toward the periphery. Numerous microtubules and microfilaments (review Chap. 2) are present in the cell processes.

SYNAPSES. A synapse is a specialized, localized region of cell contact between 2 neurons or between a neuron and its effector tissue (muscle or gland). The cell membranes of the 2 cells that are involved in a synapse do not come together completely; a 20 nm wide *synaptic gap* remains between them (Fig. 6–8).

An impulse is transmitted from one cell to the next across the synaptic gap, following the release into the synaptic gap of *neurotransmitter substances*. These substances are released from small vesicles present in the cytoplasm of the first (presynaptic) cell.

SUPPORTING CELLS. Supporting cells are not involved in impulse conduction. These cells support and nourish the neurons. Unlike the neurons, the supporting cells are capable of mitosis.

In the central nervous system the supporting cells are *glia* cells. There are several types of glia cells, with different functions. Some

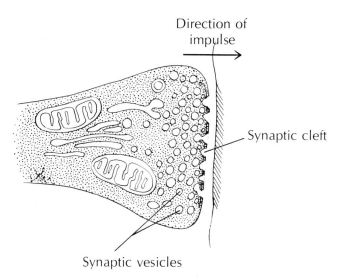

Direction of impulse

Synaptic cleft

Synaptic vesicles

Fig. 6–8. Synapse between a neuronal cell process and either another neuron or an effector tissue (a muscle cell, for example). In this diagram, the impulse travels from left to right. In the left (presynaptic) cell numerous synaptic vesicles are present. These vesicles contain the neurotransmitter substances, which are to be released in the synaptic cleft or gap in order to transmit the impulse from one cell membrane across the gap to the next cell membrane.

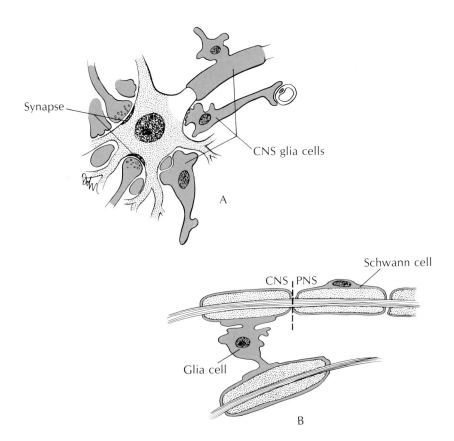

Synapse

CNS glia cells

A

Schwann cell

CNS | PNS

Glia cell

B

Fig. 6-9. A, Supporting glia cells around a multipolar neuron in the central nervous system (CNS). All nonsynaptic neuronal surfaces are covered by glia cells. In the upper right hand corner a glia cell has produced a myelin sheath around the axon. Just below it, a glia cell has cell processes, covering both a blood vessel wall (right) and part of the neuronal surface. B, Axons running from central nervous system (CNS) to peripheral nervous system (PNS). In the CNS, the axons are supported by a glia cell, whose cell processes form myelin sheaths around them. One glia cell may support several adjacent axons. In the PNS, Schwann cells support the axons, surrounding them with a myelin sheath. A Schwann cell cannot participate in the formation of more than one myelin sheath. Several Schwann cells are found along the length of an axon.

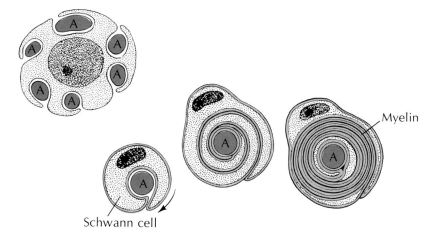

Fig. 6–10.   The relationships between axons (A) and Schwann cells is illustrated in these diagrammatic cross sections through an unmyelinated and a myelinated nerve. At left, a Schwann cell (with stippled cytoplasm) is shown, supporting several axons in depressions on its cell surface. The number of axons, thus supported, is variable. In some cases only one axon may be found in this type of relationship. No myelin sheath is formed by these Schwann cells. The 3 diagrams below show the steps in the formation of a myelin sheath around a single axon. The Schwann cell wraps itself progressively further around the axon. The concentric layers of the Schwann cell membrane, fused together, constitute the myelin sheath.

produce a sheath of fatty material, *myelin,* around the axons. Others cover the nonsynaptic surfaces of the neuronal cell bodies as well as the blood vessel walls, thereby controlling the flow of nourishment and gases to the neurons.

In the peripheral nervous system *satellite cells* cover the non-synaptic surfaces of the neuronal cell bodies in the ganglia. Schwann cells support the individual axons in the peripheral nerves. The Schwann cells in the afferent (sensory) nerves and in the efferent (somatic motor) nerves surround the axons with a sheath of myelin.

Autonomic nerves and the terminal parts of peripheral afferent and efferent nerves are unmyelinated. In these nerves Schwann cells support the axons in depressions of their cell surfaces (Figs. 6–9 and 6–10).

Organization of a Peripheral Nerve

A *nerve,* which may be identified in a gross anatomic dissection or in a histologic slide, consists of a group of axons with their supporting Schwann cells and an encapsulating frame of connective tissue with blood vessels. One axon with its associated sheath of

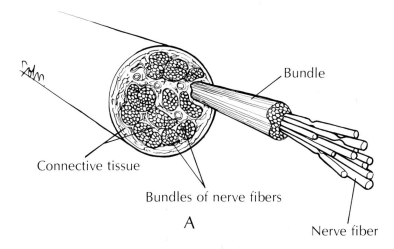

Bundle

Connective tissue

Bundles of nerve fibers

A

Nerve fiber

Fig. 6–11. A, The organization of a peripheral nerve is shown diagrammatically. The nerve is surrounded by a predominantly collagenous, connective tissue sheath. It is composed of several bundles of nerve fibers. Both bundles and individual nerve fibers are further encapsulated in connective tissue sheaths. An individual nerve fiber consists of an axon, surrounded by its sheath of Schwann cells. B, Histologic cross section through the mandibular nerve, located in the bony canal of a lower jaw. The several bundles (B) of nerve fibers, each surrounded by its connective tissue sheath, are clearly visible. The individual nerve fibers appear in cross section as tiny, open rings, some with a dot (axon) inside. The myelin is lost during histologic processing, which accounts for the seeming emptiness of the nerve fibers in histologic section. Original magnification × 10.

Schwann cells, lined up along the length of the axon, is called a *nerve fiber* (Fig. 6–11).

Let us review the differences in the use of the term *fiber* in the various tissues. In *connective tissue,* a fiber is an *inter*cellular matrix component, produced by connective tissue cells and consisting largely of proteins and some carbohydrate chains. We distinguish collagen, reticulin, elastic and oxytalan fibers. In *striated muscle,* a fiber is a large, multinucleated muscle *cell.* In a *nerve,* a fiber is a long *cell process* of a neuron (axon) with a sheath of several *supporting cells.*

Nerve Terminals

There is a variety of nerve terminals at both output and input ends of the peripheral nervous system. We will discuss here the nerve terminals of importance in the orofacial region (Fig. 6–12).

In *striated muscle,* an efferent (motor) nerve terminates on the surfaces of individual muscle cells in *motor endplates,* resembling synapses. The impulse, propagated along the nerve, is transmitted across the synaptic trough, increasing the permeability of the muscle cell membrane and touching off muscular contraction.

Within both muscles and tendons, specialized *sensory receptors* are present, feeding back information to the central nervous system about the state of contraction of the muscle and the position of the moving parts of the body.

Within the *oral mucosa* and *periodontal ligament,* 2 main types of sensory receptors should be recognized: free nerve endings and encapsulated nerve endings.

FREE NERVE ENDINGS. These are the terminal portions of afferent (sensory) axons, no longer covered by supporting Schwann cells. In the oral mucosa, such nerve endings penetrate, across the basal lamina, into the oral epithelium. These endings are generally associated with *pain* perception. Free nerve endings are also the principal sensory receptors found in the dental pulp. Toothaches are transmitted via nerves, which terminate as free nerve endings at the periphery of the dental pulp.

ENCAPSULATED NERVE ENDINGS. These consist of several terminal portions of afferent axons, surrounded by a bulbous capsule of several Schwann cells, without myelin, and some connective tissue elements. Encapsulated nerve endings are probably associated with *touch* perception. In the oral mucosa, they are highly organized *Meissner's corpuscles,* generally found in the papillary layer of the lamina propria, in some connective tissue papillae. In the periodontal ligament, the encapsulated nerve endings are small and poorly organized.

Schwann cell/Myelin sheath

A

B

Connective tissue and Schwann cells

Schwann cell

Sensory axon

C

BLOOD AND BLOOD VESSELS

In order to function and to stay alive, the cells of an organism have to be supplied constantly with all requirements for their metabolism and must be relieved of their metabolic waste products. This is a function of the *vascular system.* Other functions of this system include (1) the transport of inflammatory cells and antibodies and (2) in warm-blooded individuals, the maintenance of a constant body temperature.

The vascular system consists of a pumping organ, the *heart,* and a closed system of blood vessels, running from the heart to the organs and back to the heart. Between the heart and the organs, the blood vessels *(arteries)* branch progressively into finer vessels, until, in the organs, a network of extremely delicate vessels *(capillaries)* is formed. Between the organs and the heart, many smaller vessels combine to form progressively larger vessels *(veins),* which carry the blood back to the heart.

For tissues and organs, the essential part of the vascular system is the capillary bed, where the exchange of gases and substances occurs. The heart and the larger vessels have the role of moving the blood to and from the capillary beds.

The vascular system develops embryologically from mesenchymal cells, which form a network of delicate tubular structures, composed of the differentiated cells. These cells, *endothelial cells,* are flat (squamous), and they are arranged in an epithelium-like fashion. With further development and function, the several distinct types of blood vessels are formed, each with their characteristic wall structure. But all of the blood vessels, as well as the heart, retain an innermost lining of endothelial cells.

ARTERIES. Around the simple endothelial lining a thick layer of smooth muscle cells and elastic membranes is present. In the largest arteries, closest to the heart, there are relatively more

Fig. 6–12.   Various nerve terminals are shown diagrammatically in this figure. A, Motor endplate. The axon of a motor neuron forms a flat extension, which is located in a depression on the surface of a striated muscle fiber (stippled cytoplasm, a few myofibrils are visible). A synaptic cleft, into which the synaptic vesicles may release their neuro-transmitter substances, is present between muscle membrane and presynaptic axon membrane. B, Free nerve endings. Single sensory axons, no longer covered with Schwann cells, cross the basal lamina and terminate inside stratified squamous epithelium. C, Encapsulated nerve ending. A specific example of an encapsulated sensory terminal is illustrated: Meissner's corpuscle. It is characteristically located in a connective tissue papilla, occupying nearly all of its volume, immediately beneath the epithelium. A bulbous capsule of nonmyelinated Schwann cells and connective tissue elements surrounds the sensory axon terminals.

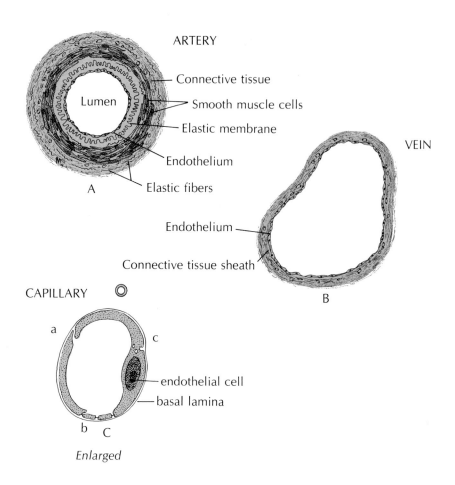

Fig. 6–13.   Diagrammatic representations of cross sections through a small artery, A, a small vein, B, and a capillary, C. The artery has a relatively cylindrical lumen, round in cross section, surrounded by a single layer of endothelial cells and a thick wall of elastic membranes, concentrically arranged smooth muscle cells and a small amount of connective tissue proper. The vein has an irregular, wide lumen, surrounded by a single layer of endothelial cells and a thin wall, consisting predominantly of connective tissue elements. A capillary, if shown proportionally, would be no larger than the small circular outline, drawn here. To show more detail, the capillary cross section is further enlarged. The capillary wall, in cross section, consists of a single endothelial cell, folded around a narrow lumen. A basal lamina is present between this cell and the surrounding tissues. a, openings at the cell junctions; b, pores; c, pinocytotic vesicles (see text for explanations).

elastic membranes (composed of elastic fibers), while in the smaller arteries, further away from the heart, there are mostly smooth muscle cells in this wall layer (Fig. 6–13, A).

The heart contracts rhythmically. If the walls of the arteries were rigid, the blood would reach the organs in squirts. In fact, when the heart contracts, the walls of the larger arteries distend and then slowly return to their original position (this is elastic rebound, a result of the action of the elastic membranes), thereby ensuring a steady flow of blood in the smaller vessels.

The contractions of smooth muscle cells in the arterial walls further aid the distribution of blood. This is particularly important in the microvascular system.

VEINS. Veins generally accompany arteries, but carry blood in the opposite direction. These vessels consist of an endothelial lining with a connective tissue reinforcement around it. Occasionally, a few smooth muscle cells are present in the walls of the largest veins. Veins contain about 70% of the total blood volume of the body at any time (Fig. 6–13, B).

CAPILLARIES. Capillaries are simple endothelial tubes approximately 5 to 7 μm in diameter. The endothelial cells and a basal lamina are the only components of a capillary wall, forming a selective barrier between the blood and the tissues. Transport across

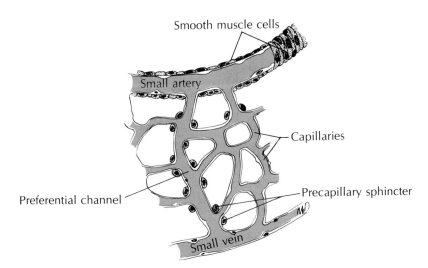

Fig. 6–14. *Simplified diagram of a microvascular bed. A small arteriole, with an inner layer of endothelial cells and a single peripheral layer of smooth muscle cells, has terminal branches, one of which is shown here, which form preferential channels to small venules (endothelial cells surrounded by a thin connective tissue sheath). From the preferential channels, several branches lead into the capillary network. At the entrance of each of these branches, a precapillary sphincter (a smooth muscle cell) is present. These sphincters control how much blood is admitted in what capillaries.*

the capillary wall may take place via (1) openings in the line of contact between adjacent endothelial cells, (2) openings across the endothelial cells, which are filled with some selective filtering material and are called *pores,* and (3) *pinocytotic vesicles,* small vesicles engulfing some material on one side of the cell, shuttling it across the cytoplasm, and releasing it at the other side of the endothelial cell (Fig. 6–13, C).

MICROVASCULATURE. Arteries and veins branch progressively into smaller blood vessels as they approach the capillary bed. The smallest arteries *(arterioles)* and the smallest veins *(venules)* form, together with the capillary bed, the microvasculature.

The terminal branch of an arteriole is called a *preferential channel,* a blood vessel leading directly to a venule. This channel has several side branches, which are entrances into the capillary bed. At any given time, most of these entrances are closed and the blood passes "by preference" through the preferential channel from the arterial side to the venous side of the microvasculature.

As may be seen in Figure 6–14, at each entrance to the capillary bed a *precapillary sphincter* is present. This sphincter consists of a smooth muscle cell, wrapped around the entrance, which by contracting closes off this entrance.

Selective, temporary occlusion of parts of the capillary bed is important. If all capillaries of the body would be open at the same time, we would not have enough blood to fill the entire vascular system and would go into *shock.* The selective opening and closing of parts of the capillary bed is presumably regulated by the specific metabolic needs of the tissue supplied by the capillary bed.

BLOOD AND BLOOD CELLS

Blood consists of two component parts, a liquid phase *(plasma)* and a cellular phase *(blood cells).* Blood *serum* is blood plasma from which certain clotting factors, especially fibrinogen, have been removed. *Blood cells* comprise about 45% of the total blood volume. A listing of the characteristics of the cells found in circulating blood is presented here.

The cellular phase of blood can be subdivided into 3 main groups (Fig. 6–15):

I *Red cells* (erythrocytes)

II *White cells* (leukocytes)
    A.   Granular leukocytes
        1. Neutrophils
        2. Eosinophils
        3. Basophils
    B.   Nongranular leukocytes
        1. Monocytes
        2. Lymphocytes

III *Platelets*

Fig. 6–15.   Normal white blood cells (leukocytes), photographed in a surrounding of red blood cells (erythrocytes). A, Neutrophil (polymorphonuclear leukocyte). B, Neutrophil. C, Eosinophil. D, Basophil. E, Monocyte. F, Monocyte. (From Wintrobe, M.M., et al.: Clinical Hematology. 7th Ed. Philadelphia, Lea & Febiger, 1974.)

Red Cells (Erythrocytes)

The cytoplasm of these cells is filled with hemoglobin (which binds oxygen). The hemoglobin gives the cells their red color, which in turn is responsible for the red color of the blood. The red cells have no nucleus, it is lost during cell development.

Function: transport of O_2 and facilitation of transport of CO_2.
Size: 7 μm
Prevalence: 4 to 6 million/mm³ of blood
 in men the average is 5.7 million/mm³
 in women the average is 4.5 million/mm³
Where formed: red bone marrow
Where destroyed: red bone marrow and spleen
Survival time in circulating blood: about 120 days

White Cells (Leukocytes)

Prevalence: 5000 to 10,000/mm³ blood

Granular Leukocytes

The cytoplasm of all granular leukocytes is filled with distinctive granules, seen in the light microscope. These granules are lysosomes, filled with specific enzymes. In addition, the granular leukocytes have characteristic nuclei.

Where formed: red bone marrow
Where destroyed: connective tissue; alimentary tract; lungs
Survival time: unknown; estimated between 1 day and 2 weeks.

 NEUTROPHIL (polymorphonuclear leukocyte). This is an ameboid cell. The nucleus has several lobes. The granules contain mostly lysosomal, proteolytic enzymes. The granules are neither acid nor alkaline, reacting in neutral fashion with the histologic stains.

Function: first defense against bacterial invasion, *phagocytosis.*
Size: 11 μm
Prevalence: 60% of all leukocytes

 EOSINOPHIL. This is a somewhat ameboid cell. The nucleus has 2 lobes. The cytoplasm contains large alkaline granules, staining preferentially with eosin. These granules contain specific lysosomal enzymes.

Function: defense against strange proteins; involvement in allergy reaction.
Size: 12 μm
Prevalence: 2% of all leukocytes

 BASOPHIL. This is a strongly ameboid cell. The nucleus is bent in a U-shape or S-shape. This nucleus is barely visible due to the presence of large acid granules in the cytoplasm. These granules

stain preferentially with the base hematoxyline. They contain histamine and perhaps heparin (vaso-active substances).
Function: Release of granular material in the presence of an antigen (?).
Size: 10 μm
Prevalence: 0.5% of all leukocytes

Nongranular Leukocytes

MONOCYTE. This cell does *not* have specific granules in the cytoplasm. In the mature cell, the nucleus is placed in a somewhat eccentric position and is kidney-shaped.
Function: becomes a macrophage in connective tissue.
Size: 17 μm
Prevalence: 3 to 8% of all leukocytes
Survival time: circulates in blood 1 to 2 days; *months* in tissues.
Where formed: red bone marrow
Where destroyed: tissue
LYMPHOCYTE. No specific granules are present in the cytoplasm of this cell type. In small lymphocytes the nucleus fills most of the cell.
Function: promotes phagocytosis and produces antibodies (cellular and humoral defense)
Size: 6 to 8 μm (small); 12 to 15 μm (large)
Prevalence: 25 to 33% of all leukocytes
Where formed: bone marrow and lymphoid tissues
Where destroyed: spleen
Survival time: unknown, variable.

Platelets

Platelets are cell fragments of a specific cell type in red bone marrow (megakaryocyte). They have no nuclei.
Function: promote blood clotting
Size: 2 to 3 μm
Prevalence: 300,000/mm³
Where formed: red bone marrow
Where destroyed: blood clot
Survival time: unknown

LYMPHATICS

Lymphatic Vessels

Soon after the blood enters a capillary bed, a number of substances, including fluid from the blood plasma, passes through the capillary walls into the surrounding tissues. This movement out of the capillaries is due largely to the hydrostatic pressure that is built up in the arteries on the arterial side of the microvasculature. Since larger molecules, particularly albumin, cannot pass through the capillary walls, the concentration of these molecules increases in the blood remaining in the capillaries, which is now also reduced in fluid volume.

Because of the distribution of the remaining blood over many small capillaries, the hydrostatic pressure is decreased in those vessels and the movement of fluid and substances out of the capillaries stops. However, because of the high concentration of the larger molecules in the blood, some of the fluid that did move out of the capillaries is now attracted back into the blood stream (by a process of osmosis).

Usually, not all fluid returns to the capillaries in this manner, and so the tissues need another mechanism to remove the fluid that is left behind. The needed mechanism is provided by the *lymphatic vessels*.

Lymphatic capillaries run parallel with the blood capillaries. Lymphatic capillaries consist, as do blood capillaries, of endothelial cells, but there is no clear basal lamina around the vessels, and large openings are present between the endothelial cells. Thus, there is easy access for fluid and substances from the tissues into the lymphatic capillaries. Lymphatic vessels do *not* carry anything *to* the tissues. They only carry material, mostly fluid or *lymph,* away *from* the tissues.

A system of increasingly larger lymphatic vessels collects the contents of the smaller lymphatic capillaries, and finally the lymph is returned to the blood stream, just before it returns to the heart.

In addition to the surplus of the fluid that had moved out of the blood capillaries and did not move back into these capillaries, the lymphatic vessels occasionally carry other matter away from the tissues. This becomes particularly important when these tissues are diseased. Breakdown products resulting from inflammations or metastatic cells from malignant tumors may be carried from their original location to other parts of the body via the lymphatic vessels.

Some safeguards against such components are provided by the presence of small organs, *lymph nodes,* which are found along the lymphatic pathways. These nodes consist of an encapsulated mass of lymphoid tissue (p. 130) and serve, not always perfectly, as filters of the lymph. Several lymphatic vessels, arriving at the outside surface of a lymph node, break up into a capillary network inside the node, and after this passage, during which the extraneous matter has been removed and digested by the cells of the lymphoid tissue, the capillaries come together again into one large lymphatic vessel. This carries the filtered lymph away from the lymph node.

In healthy individuals, lymph nodes are inconspicuous, but in disease, when the nodes are actively performing filtering functions,

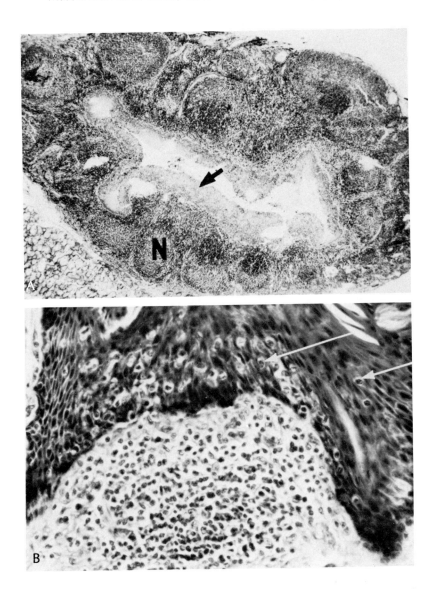

Fig. 6–16.   A, Histologic cross section through a deep pit (crypt) in a human tonsil. The crypt is lined with stratified squamous epithelium (arrow). Lymphoid tissue is arranged underneath the epithelium. Some accumulations of the darkly staining lymphocytes, lymphatic nodules (N), are visible in the lymphoid tissue. No clear connective tissue capsule surrounds the tonsillar tissue. Original magnification × 10. B, Stratified squamous epithelial lining of a human tonsillar crypt. Several lymphocytes (arrows) have invaded the epithelium and are located among the epithelial cells. Original magnification × 100.

they become swollen and painful. Diagnostically, such nodes are important. They may indicate the presence of an inflammation or the spread of a malignant tumor. A gross anatomy atlas should be used to help you to locate the lymph nodes critical to the orofacial area.

Lymph Nodes

Lymph nodes are lymphoid organs. They consist of an encapsulated mass of lymphoid tissue. Lymphoid tissue is a specialized, reticular loose connective tissue, consisting of reticular cells in intimate relation with a delicate network of reticulin fibers, in which accumulations of lymphocytes are present. These accumulations are called lymphatic nodules, and they are areas where lymphocytes are actively proliferating. The lymphocytes are capable of developing specific immune defenses against any foreign material that might pass through the lymph nodes. In addition, macrophages are present in lymph nodes capable of phagocytosis of any undesired foreign matter.

As already noted, one of the clinically important functions of the lymph nodes is the filtering of the lymph passing through these nodes.

Tonsils

Tonsils are special lymphoid organs, located around the passageway between oral cavity and pharynx. These organs consist of lymphoid tissue, which is arranged underneath and around deep grooves and pits, formed by the oral and pharyngeal epithelium into this tissue.

Many lymphocytes are located in all layers of the epithelium. The tonsils may be thought of as an early warning system, which serves to detect the nature of the substances, entering the body via the digestive tract, and to prepare an early immune defense against any dangerous substances (Fig. 6–16).

In contrast with the lymph nodes, tonsils have *only* lymphatic vessels at their periphery, which carry lymph and lymphocytes away from the tonsil. Frequently, tonsils are not well separated from the underlying connective tissue by a dense fibrous capsule. As a result, surgical removal of these organs is difficult.

SELECTED READING LIST

Muscle Tissue

Bloom, W., and Fawcett, D.W.: Muscular tissue. In *A Textbook of Histology.* 10th Ed. Philadelphia, W.B. Saunders Co., 1975.
Huxley, H.E.: The mechanism of muscular contraction. Science, *164*:1356, 1969.

Nervous Tissue

Copenhaver, W.M., Bunge, R.P., and Bunge, M.B.: Organization of nervous tissue. In *Bailey's Textbook of Histology*. 16th Ed. Baltimore, Williams & Wilkins, 1971.

Gauthier, G.F.: The motor end-plate. In *The Peripheral Nerve*. Edited by D.N. Landon. London, Chapman and Hall, 1976.

Grossman, R.C., and Hattis, B.F.: Oral mucosal sensory innervation and sensory experience: a review. In *Symposium on Oral Sensation and Perception*. Edited by J.F. Bosma, Springfield, Ill., Charles C Thomas, 1967.

Katz, B.: *Nerve, Muscle and Synapse*. New York, McGraw-Hill Book Co., 1966.

Noback, C. R., and Demarest, R. J.: *The Nervous System: Introduction and Review*. New York, McGraw-Hill Book Co., 1972.

Pappas, G.D., and Waxman, S.G.: Synaptic fine structure—morphological correlates of chemical and electrotonic transmission. In *Structure and Function of Synapses*. Edited by G.D. Pappas and D.P. Purpura. New York, Raven Press, 1972.

Blood, Blood Vessels, Lymphatics

DiFiore, M.S.H.: *Atlas of Human Histology*. 3rd Ed. Philadelphia, Lea & Febiger, 1967.

Lavelle, C.L.B.: The blood supply of the oral tissues. In *Applied Physiology of the Mouth*. Edited by C.L.B. Lavelle. Bristol, John Wright and Sons, 1975.

Weiss, L.: *The Cells and Tissues of the Immune System*. Englewood Cliffs, N.J. Prentice-Hall, 1972.

Wickramasinghe, S.N.: *Human Bone Marrow*. Oxford, Blackwell Scientific Publications, 1975.

Williams, W.J., Beutler, E., Erslaw, A.J., and Rundles, R.W.: *Hematology*. New York, McGraw-Hill Book Co., 1972.

Wintrobe, M.M. et al.: Clinical Hematology. 7th Ed., Philadelphia, Lea & Febiger, 1974.

Zweifach, B.W.: *Functional Behavior of the Microcirculation*. Springfield, Ill., Charles C Thomas, 1961.

Zweifach, B.W.: Microcirculation. Ann. Rev. Physiol., *35*:117, 1973.

Chapter 7

EMBRYOLOGIC DEVELOPMENT OF THE FACE AND ORAL CAVITY

The human body consists of many groups of specialized cells forming tissues, organs and organ systems. In this chapter we will give a brief description of some of the developmental events transforming one single cell (the *fertilized ovum*) into a human body. Special emphasis will be placed on the development of the facial region.

Many stages of embryologic development require complex interactions and differentiations of cells. If there is any disturbance in the normal sequence of events, especially during the first 3 months of pregnancy, a *malformation* is likely to result. Such malformations, which are evident at birth, are called *congenital* malformations.

As a dental health professional, you must be concerned about congenital malformations in at least 2 situations:

1. Congenital malformations of the head and neck region occur in about 1 out of every 700 live births. The chances that you will treat patients who were born with such malformations are real. These malformations may range from serious clefts in the face and/or palate to small deficiencies of the soft palate or cysts underneath an otherwise intact oral mucosa. It is hoped that such patients will have undergone surgical treatment for these defects by the time they seek your professional service. However, in the more serious cases, special consideration and adaptation of your treatment still may be necessary.

2. Certain congenital malformations, such as facial or palatal clefts, may be related to "environmental" conditions, for example, the use of certain drugs by pregnant women during susceptible stages of their pregnancy. Women in the first 3 months of pregnancy are particularly vulnerable in this respect. Treatment of such patients must be directed toward prevention of congenital malformations.

In human prenatal development, 3 distinct periods may be distinguished (Fig. 7–1).

Fig. 7–1.   Conditions at the beginning and end of each of the 3 distinct periods in human prenatal development. The first period begins with the newly fertilized ovum and ends with the attachment of the conceptus to the wall of the uterus. The second or embryonic period begins with the small vesicle of the conceptus attaching to the wall of the uterus and ends with an individual of recognizably human appearance. The third, or fetal, period begins with the small, but recognizably human, fetus and ends with the newborn baby.

1. *THE FIRST WEEK* (the period of the *unattached concep-tus*). In this week the fertilized ovum travels from the site where it was fertilized to the womb (uterus) and becomes attached to the wall of this organ by the end of the first week. At that time, a number of changes have occurred, which have transformed the single cell into a vesicle, consisting of a layer of peripheral cells and a small accumulation of embryonic cells.

2. *THE EMBRYONIC PERIOD* (the second through eighth week). In this time most organ systems and organs of the future individual are formed. This is a period of *differentiation,* and most congenital malformations develop at this time. At the end of the embryonic period, the developing individual has a recognizably human appearance.

3. *THE FETAL PERIOD* (the third through the ninth month). This is predominantly a time of *growth* of existing structures and will not be further described in this chapter. By the end of the fourth month, the physician is able to detect the fetal heartbeat, and only some weeks later the pregnant woman is able to feel the movements of the fetus (quickening).

FERTILIZATION

Human development begins when one female germ cell and one male germ cell unite. This is fertilization.

The female germ cell, the *ovum,* develops in 1 of the 2 ovaries of a woman. Once a month, during the period between puberty and menopause, an ovum is released from 1 of the ovaries. This process is called ovulation. Ovulation takes place 14 days before the next expected menstrual period. Following ovulation, an ovum survives for about 24 hours in the female genital tract. The ovum is normally swept into the *uterine tube* and moved along the tube toward the uterus.

The male germ cell, the *sperm,* develops in 1 of the 2 testes of a man. Generally, sperm production is continuous from puberty until death. During sexual intercourse 300 to 500 million sperms are deposited in the vagina near the uterus. The sperms begin to move into the uterus and the uterine tubes at a considerable speed. The survival time of these germ cells in the female genital tract is 3 to 4 days.

About 10 hours after intercourse, 300 to 500 sperms have traveled two-thirds the length of the uterine tube. *If a living ovum is present at that time* in the tube, one of these germ cells will unite with the ovum (fertilization) and prenatal development begins (Fig. 7–2). (*Note:* Each germ cell contains only one-half the normal number of chromosomes in their nucleus [23 chromosomes instead of 46]. During fertilization the nuclei of both germ cells are

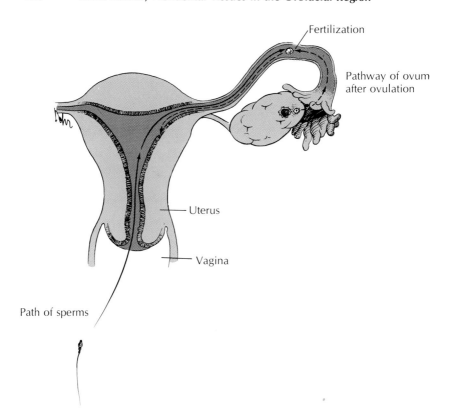

Fig. 7–2.   Pathways of ovum and sperms before and immediately after fertilization. The ovum, released from one of the ovaries, is swept into the uterine tube and is moved through the tube in the direction of the uterus (broken line). The sperms, deposited in the vagina, move through the uterus and up into the uterine tube (solid line). One sperm cell is illustrated, disproportionately large. The size of the projectile-shaped cell body of this cell is about 1/20 that of an ovum. The length of the long tail, used to propel the sperm cell into the uterine tube, is about 1/2 the diameter of an ovum. In the uterine tube one sperm cell fertilizes the ovum. The fertilized ovum is moved slowly (broken line) from the site of fertilization toward the uterus, where it becomes attached to the uterine wall.

combined, restoring the number of chromosomes to 46—23 from the male and 23 from the female parent.)

THE FIRST WEEK

While the ovum is traveling to the uterus, following fertilization, it undergoes a series of mitotic divisions (Fig. 7–3).

On the *fourth day* after fertilization, the structure, consisting of 16 to 32 cells, enters the cavity of the uterus. On the *fifth day* a central cavity develops inside this previously solid mass of cells. The

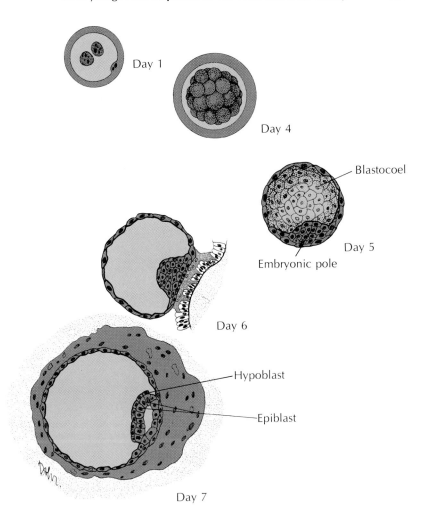

Fig. 7–3. The appearance of the human conceptus during the first week of prenatal development. On day 1, the day of fertilization, the nucleus of the sperm cell is about to fuse with the nucleus of the ovum, thus restoring the chromosome number to 46. On day 4 the conceptus still moves about freely. The number of cells has increased from 1 to 16 by a few mitoses. The size of the conceptus, however, has barely increased. On day 5 the membrane, which surrounded the ovum and later the conceptus, has been lost. A central cavity (blastocoel) has developed. There is a distinct, single layer of peripheral cells and an accumulation of cells at the embryonic pole. The conceptus is called a blastocyst and is shown diagrammatically (cut open) to reveal its 3-dimensional structure. On day 6 the conceptus becomes attached to the wall of the uterus. The first attachment site is the embryonic pole. On day 7 the conceptus becomes further attached and embedded (implanted) in the uterine wall. In the cell-accumulation at the embryonic pole, 2 distinct layers of cells are becoming visible: an epiblast layer and a hypoblast layer. Between epiblast and peripheral cell layers a second cavity is forming. Epiblast and hypoblast now constitute a clearly delineated embryonic disc.

structure now develops into a *blastocyst,* which consists of a single layer of peripheral cells surrounding a fluid-filled cavity (blastocoel). At one site the cellular layer is thicker, because of the presence of about 8 slightly larger cells. The site is called the *embryonic pole,* and the larger cells will give rise to the actual embryo, which later becomes the fetus. The smaller peripheral cells give rise to most of the fetal membranes that will surround the developing individual (Fig. 7–3).

On the *sixth day* the developing structure, or conceptus, begins to attach to the wall of the uterus and *implantation* begins. This is essential for the success of the pregnancy, since implantation ensures the development of the placenta, which is necessary for the interaction between fetal and maternal circulation. The conceptus slowly invades the uterine tissues to some depth and, by the end of the second week, it is completely surrounded by these tissues.

On the *seventh day* the actual embryonic cells begin to form 2 distinct cell layers.

THE EMBRYONIC PERIOD

During this period, the second, third and fourth weeks of development have distinct characteristics.

1. *THE SECOND WEEK.* During the second week the process of implantation continues. By further mitoses and differentiation, the actual embryonic cells have formed 2 distinct cell layers (Fig. 7–4, A): *epiblast,* facing the peripheral cell layer, and *hypoblast,* facing the fluid-filled blastocoel cavity. Between epiblast and peripheral cells a second cavity, the *amniotic cavity,* forms. Epiblast and hypoblast now constitute a clearly separate *disc* 2 cell layers thick, suspended between 2 fluid-filled cavities. This disc will give rise to the embryo and is therefore called the *embryonic disc.*

For the sake of simplicity, we will not discuss here the further development of the fetal membranes, placenta, yolk sac and umbilical cord. The interested reader is referred to the standard texts of human embryology. The descriptions in this chapter will be limited to the fate of the embryonic disc.

2. *THE THIRD WEEK.* This week is characterized by the establishment of a rod-shaped thickening on the epiblast surface of the embryonic disc. This thickening is called the *primitive streak,* and it is the first external manifestation of the long axis of the future human body. We can now visualize a *bilateral symmetry* in the disc, as well as a head (cephalic) end and tail (caudal) end (Fig. 7–4).

Continued proliferation of epiblast cells now produces a wave-like movement of these cells *toward* the primitive streak. At the primitive streak many epiblast cells move "downward" to a posi-

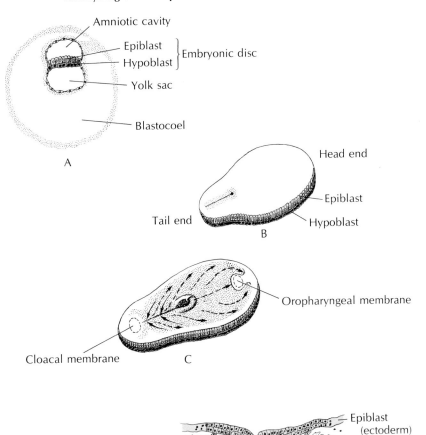

Fig. 7–4. *Developments in the second week, A, and third week, B–D, of human prenatal development are shown diagrammatically. A, During the second week the epiblast and hypoblast are clearly defined within the embryonic disc. The second cavity, formed between epiblast and peripheral cells, becomes clearly established as the amniotic cavity. An outgrowth of hypoblast cells.lines a yolk sac, thus subdividing the blastocoel cavity. In the following diagrams only the structures of the embryonic disc have been depicted in 3 dimensions. B, The embryonic disc seen from "above" (epiblast side) at the beginning of the third week. A central thickening, the primitive streak, has formed at the tail end of the epiblast layer. C, Several epiblast cells, while undergoing further mitoses, move to the primitive streak (solid arrows), where they descend to a position between epiblast and hypoblast layers and establish a middle layer (broken arrows). This third (middle) layer is formed everywhere in the embryonic disc, except in the areas of oropharyngeal and cloacal membranes, which continue to consist of only 2 cell layers. D, A diagrammatic section through the embryonic disc, at the level of the primitive streak, shows the movement of the epiblast cells. Most of these cells form the mesoderm. Some cells become inserted in the hypoblast layer, which now becomes the endoderm. The remainder of the epiblast layer becomes the ectoderm.*

tion between the epiblast and hypoblast layers, and they migrate between these 2 layers. The migrating cells establish a *middle layer*, which is sandwiched between epiblast and hypoblast. This middle layer is present in all parts of the embryo, except in 2 small, circular regions, the *oropharyngeal membrane* and the *cloacal membrane*. These membranes continue to consist of 2 cell layers only, and they represent the beginning and end points of the future digestive tract.

By the end of the third week, the embryonic disc consists of 3 distinct layers *(germ layers)* (Fig. 7–5): *ectoderm*, from the original epiblast, *mesoderm* (the *new* layer, between ectoderm and endoderm), derived from epiblast cells that have moved down through the primitive streak, and *endoderm*, derived in part from the original hypoblast and in part from *some* epiblast cells, which moved down through the primitive streak and pushed into the original hypoblast layer. The cells in each of these 3 germ layers have already undergone certain differentiations, which make them different from the cells in the other 2 germ layers.

It is now possible to give, in general outline, a list of tissues and organs in the human body and to indicate from which of these 3 germ layers each is derived.

Table 7–1 is a *general* outline of the derivatives of the 3 germ layers. Some additional information is needed for the consideration of the derivatives in the facial region (see p. 141).

3. *THE FOURTH WEEK.* During the fourth week of development, the formation of the central nervous system is initiated. The central nervous system is derived from cells that are located in a thickened central band of ectoderm *(neurectoderm),* running from the cephalic to the caudal end of the embryonic disc.

This thickened band, or *neural plate*, is first folded into a *neural groove*, which subsequently closes to become a *neural tube*. During the closure of the neural tube, the adjacent ectoderm grows over it and covers it. The closed neural tube lies, therefore, in mesoderm.

Ectoderm
Neurectoderm
Mesoderm
Endoderm

Fig. 7–5. Simplified, diagrammatic, transverse section through the embryonic disc, which consists of 3 germ layers by the end of the third week. The key to the right indicates the ectoderm, mesoderm, and endoderm. A small, central strip of ectoderm will differentiate further into neurectoderm, which will form the central nervous system.

Table 7–1. Derivatives of 3 Germ Layers

Germ Layer	Derivatives

Ectoderm	Nerve tissue (from neurectoderm)
	Epithelium
	    Oral epithelium
	    Epidermis

Mesoderm	Connective tissues
	    Connective tissue proper
	    Skeletal tissue (bone, cartilage)
	    Circulatory system (heart, blood, blood vessels)
	    Lymphatics
	Muscle tissue
	    Heart
	    Striated muscle
	    Smooth muscle
	Urinary system
	    Epithelium
	    Connective tissue

Endoderm	Epithelial lining of digestive tract (except oral cavity) Epithelial lining of respiratory tract

Closure of the neural tube occurs first in the neck region of the embryo and then continues, in a zipper-like fashion, in the direction of both the head and the tail (Fig. 7–6).

During closure of the neural tube, 2 peripheral strips of neurectoderm, the *neural crest,* become separated from the neural tube, but are covered over by ectoderm as well. The cells of those 2 strips, which come to lie on either side of the neural tube, will eventually migrate to many regions of the body, where they will differentiate into many different types of cells. Important to this discussion is the fact that these cells will become ganglion cells (both sensory and autonomic) and melanocytes.

In the *facial region* the *neural crest cells* migrate *among* the already present mesoderm cells, where they further differentiate and give rise to several tissues: (1) bone and cartilage, (2) connective tissue proper, and (3) some dental tissues (dental pulp and dentin, cementum and periodontal ligament). The *mesoderm* in the facial region gives rise to (1) blood vessels, and (2) muscle tissue.

Please *note* that the facial region is an *exceptional* region. In the rest of the body, neural crest cells do *not* differentiate into bone, cartilage or connective tissue cells and *certainly not* into cells that form dental tissues.

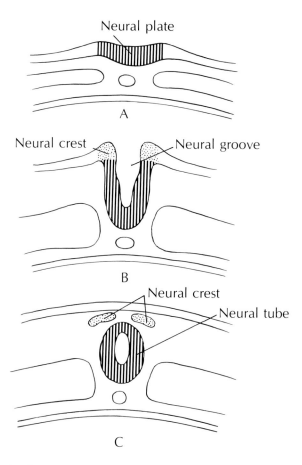

Fig. 7–6. *The development of the central nervous system during the fourth week of prenatal development. A, B, and C represent chronologically sequential cross sections through the embryonic disc. A, A central strip of ectoderm, neurectoderm, has thickened into a neural plate. B, The neural plate has become folded into a neural groove. The 2 strips of neural crest (stippled) are clearly visible. C, The neural groove has closed into a neural tube. The neural tube and the 2 strips of neural crest are covered over by ectoderm.*

Folding and Curving of the Embryo

In the foregoing discussion, we have considered the embryo as a flat disc consisting of 3 distinct cell layers (except in the areas of the oropharyngeal and cloacal membranes, which consist of 2 cell layers). Actually, the flat embryonic disc is transformed during the third and fourth weeks of development into a curved, tubular structure, as the result of flexions and foldings (Fig. 7–7).

As a result of these events, the ectoderm comes to lie on the outside of the tubular structure and the endoderm on the inside. The foldings are produced by the extensive growth of both ectoderm and central nervous system, compared with the much slower growth of the endoderm. The faster growing regions, therefore, have to "bulge" out of the way (Fig. 7–8).

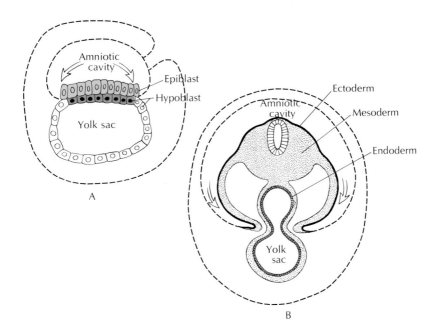

Fig. 7–7. *Transformation of the flat embryonic disc at the beginning of the third week, A, to a tubular structure at the end of the fourth week, B, of development, seen in cross sections. During this period of folding, the ectoderm comes to lie on the outside of the embryo, while the endoderm is gradually enclosed at the inside, becoming the lining of the digestive and respiratory tracts. The arrows indicate the direction in which the amniotic cavity is enlarged, until it finally almost completely surrounds the embryo (later the fetus). Concurrently with the enlargement of the amniotic cavity, the blastocoel cavity becomes reduced in size and finally disappears.*

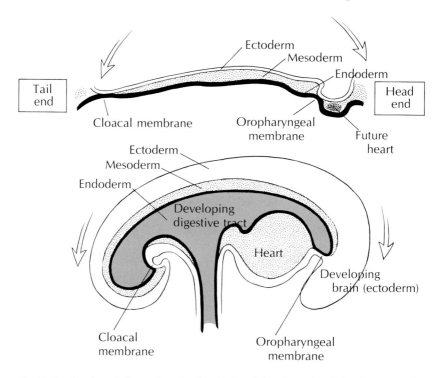

Fig. 7–8. Curving of the embryo in the third and fourth weeks of development. The embryonic disc is shown in a section along its entire length (top figure). The 3 germ layers are illustrated. Cloacal and oropharyngeal membranes consist of 2 germ layers. The amniotic cavity (on the ectoderm side) enlarges in the direction of the arrows. Since the ectoderm (which includes the central nervous system in this diagram) grows much more extensively than the endoderm, the embryo becomes curved, with ectoderm at the larger, bulging side (bottom figure).

The Facial Region

Development of the facial region begins in the fourth week of prenatal life and is completed during the twelfth week (remember that the fetal period begins after 8 weeks). However, the most critical events in the development of the face take place *before* the fetal period begins.

In the fourth week of development, the rapidly growing brain bulges over the oropharyngeal membrane. The latter is disintegrating, establishing access into the digestive tract from the amniotic cavity (Fig. 7–9). The area of the future face is squeezed between the brain and the heart. A bulging strand of tissue runs between the forebrain region and the developing heart, on either side of the distintegrating oropharyngeal membrane. This is called the *mandibular arch.*

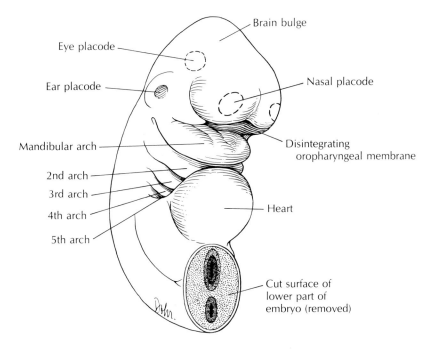

Fig. 7–9.   *Three-dimensional diagram of the upper part of a human embryo at about 4 weeks of prenatal development. The cut surface, where the lower part of the embryo has been removed, is shown. The facial region is located between the bulge of the developing forebrain and the large developing heart. Five pairs of swellings (mandibular or first arch and second through fifth arches) are illustrated in the neck region of the embryo. Between mandibular arch and bulging forebrain is the primitive oral cavity. At this location, the oropharyngeal membrane is disintegrating, establishing an open connection between amniotic cavity and primitive gut. The organs of special sense are represented at this stage by rounded placodes of thickened ectoderm. There are 3 pairs of these placodes: nasal, eye and ear placodes.*

The mandibular arch is the first of 5 pairs of swellings (the 4 others are indicated in Figure 7–9 as the second through the fifth arches). The 4 other pairs of swellings are involved predominantly in the formation of the neck region. The organization of the skeletal elements in the adult neck is a reflection of this original, *segmental* organization in arches.

However, for the development of the face proper, only the first or mandibular arch will be considered, in addition to the swelling of the tissues over the brain: the so-called *frontonasal process*.

In the adult face, the parts formed by the tissues of the frontonasal process are (1) the forehead, and (2) the nose. The parts, formed by the tissues of the mandibular arch, are (1) the midface, without the nose, and (2) the lower face (Fig. 7–10).

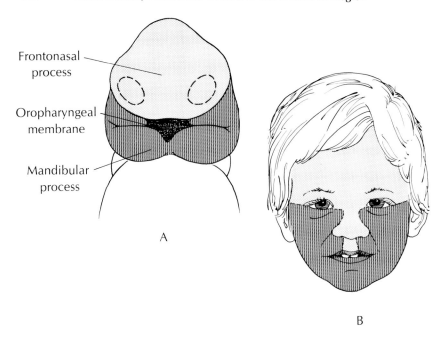

Fig. 7–10.   The facial region of a 4-week-old human embryo, **A,** *and of a young child,* **B,** *are shown, seen from front. The lightly stippled frontonasal process in* **A** *will give rise to forehead, nose and midsection of upper lip, similarly stippled in* **B.** *The mandibular arch, darkly shaded in* **A,** *will give rise to a large part of the midface and all of the lower face, similarly shaded in* **B.**

The development of the face is best considered as the forward growth, around nasal and oral cavities, of a number of swellings or *processes* arising from the frontonasal process and the mandibular arch. These swellings have a core of mesenchyme, derived from neural crest cells and mesoderm cells, and an outer covering of ectoderm.

DEVELOPMENT OF THE NOSE. The nasal epithelium, for the sensation of smell in the fully formed individual, is present on the surface of the frontonasal process of the embryo in the form of 2 *nasal placodes.* Placodes are rounded areas of specialized thickened ectoderm, which is comparable to the neurectoderm of the neural plate. Placodes are found at the locations of developing *organs* of *special sense*—eyes, ears and nose. The nasal placodes will develop into olfactory epithelium.

Parts of the frontonasal process begin to swell around these nasal placodes. The placodes themselves do not grow forward, while the surrounding swellings do. As the result of this uneven growth, the nasal placodes stay behind and come to lie in deep pits, the future nasal cavities.

The swellings around these pits, all derived from the frontonasal process, are identified as 2 *lateral nasal* processes and 2 *medial nasal* processes. The lateral nasal processes form the sides of the nose, while the medial nasal processes form the bridge of the nose and the philtrum of the upper lip (Fig. 7–11).

DEVELOPMENT OF THE MIDDLE AND LOWER FACE. The lower face is formed directly by the bilateral swellings *(mandibular processes)* of the mandibular arch. The middle face is formed by a pair of separate swellings *(maxillary* processes) which develop on the upper surfaces of the mandibular processes.

Each maxillary process rapidly grows forward between lateral nasal process and mandibular process, and then makes contact with the lower edge of the medial nasal process (Fig. 7–12).

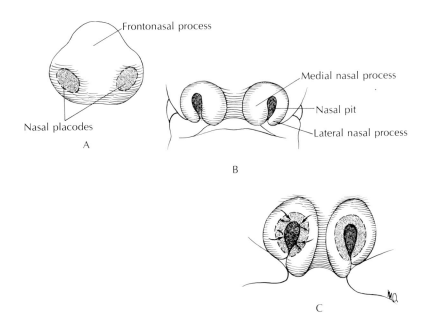

Fig. 7–11. A, *The nasal placodes are still located on the ectodermal surface of the frontonasal process (at 4 weeks of development). The nasal placodes do not grow forward as much as the surrounding tissues. As a result, at a slightly later stage, B, the nasal placodes have stayed behind and are now located in nasal pits, surrounded by several swellings (lateral nasal and medial nasal processes), which have developed from the frontonasal process. In C, the situation in the 6th week of development, the placodes are lying deeper in the nasal pits, which are in contact with the primitive oral cavity below. The lateral nasal processes will form the sides of the nose. The medial nasal processes will form the bridge of the nose and the central strip of the upper lip.*

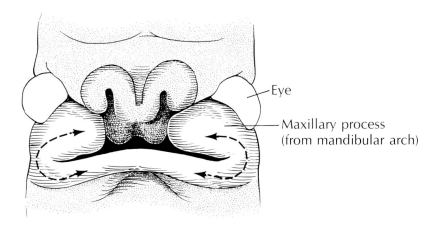

Eye

Maxillary process
(from mandibular arch)

Fig. 7–12. *Contributions to the development of the face by components of the mandibular arch during the fifth and sixth weeks of development. The mandibular arch will form the lower face directly, by further increase in size. In addition, 2 maxillary processes will form as additional swellings on the upper surfaces of the mandibular arch and will give rise to a large part of the midface. The maxillary processes grow forward (2 top arrows), first establishing contact with the lateral nasal processes and subsequently with the medial nasal processes.*

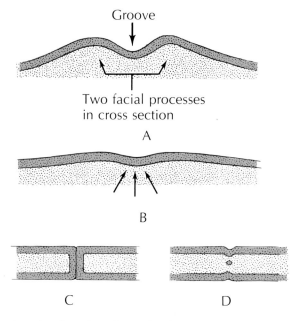

Groove

Two facial processes
in cross section

A

B

C   D

Fig. 7–13. *A section through 2 adjacent facial processes (swellings) and an intervening groove are shown diagrammatically in A and B. During normal development the groove is eliminated by increased tissue growth in the groove region. When two epithelially covered processes meet each other across a space (as happens in the development of the definitive palate), the epithelia of the 2 processes fuse (illustrated in a diagrammatic section through such processes in C). Subsequently, the epithelium in the fusion seam is broken down and continuity is established between the mesenchymal cores of the 2 processes, D.*

Initially, grooves of various depths separate the facial processes from each other. Required for the *normal* development of the face are (1) correlated speed and amounts of forward growth of the various facial processes, and (2) elimination of the grooves between the processes. On the external surface of the face, grooves between adjacent facial processes are eliminated by the proliferation of the mesenchyme underneath the ectoderm lining the deepest part of the groove. Because of this proliferation, the groove area "catches up" with the forward growth of the facial processes and the groove is eliminated (Fig. 7–13, A, B). If a groove is not eliminated, or is partially eliminated, a *facial cleft* may result. Facial clefts may be complete or incomplete; bilateral or unilateral (Figs. 7–14 and 7–15).

TIMETABLE. The groove in the future chin area, between the 2 mandibular processes, is the first to be eliminated at about 4 weeks. The grooves between maxillary and medial nasal processes are the last to be eliminated, at about 6 weeks.

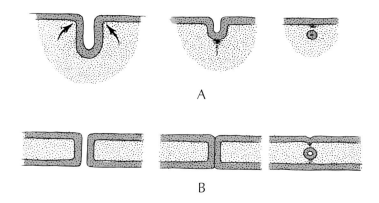

A

B

Fig. 7–14.   A *in this figure should be compared with* A *and* B *in Fig. 7–13:* B *should be compared with* C *and* D *in Fig. 7–13.* A, *Several possible failures in the elimination of a groove between 2 adjacent facial processes are illustrated. In the left diagram, the facial processes have grown forward, but the groove area has not grown much if at all. In such a case a complete facial cleft results. In the middle diagram, some groove elimination has taken place, but a small part of the groove persists. This results in an incomplete facial cleft. In the right diagram, the groove has been eliminated, but some epithelium was pinched off and has remained in the mesenchyme. Such an epithelial remnant may enlarge and develop into a developmental cyst in postnatal life.* B, *Failures in the fusion between 2 epithelially covered processes, which approach each other across an open space, are illustrated. In the left diagram, the facial processes remain too short and never touch. This results in a complete cleft. In the middle diagram, the facial processes touch, but the epithelial seam is not broken down. During further development such processes may be pulled apart and a complete cleft may result. In the right diagram, some epithelium has been broken down after fusion, but a large remnant remains. This remnant may be large enough to form a submucous cleft or it may develop into a cyst.*

Fig. 7–15. In this diagram of a face, the broken lines indicate the possible locations of facial clefts, formed if any of the events shown in Figure 7–14A occur in any of these locations. The areas between the broken lines correspond with the areas formed by the original facial processes.

DEVELOPMENT OF THE PALATE. By the age of 6 weeks, the external face of the embryo has begun to assume human features. In the deepest parts of the nasal pits tissues have degenerated, creating an opening between nasal and oral cavities. Thus, there is an open connection between the primitive nasal cavities and oral cavity. The strand of tissue running horizontally in front of this open connection, between the oral cavity and the two nasal cavities, is the *primitive palate.* It is formed by the combined medial nasal processes and a small part of both maxillary processes. This becomes the upper lip and the frontal part of the alveolar arch of the upper jaw (incisor region). What remains to be formed is the *definitive palate:* most of the hard palate and all of the soft palate, and these are formed between weeks 6 and 12 of prenatal development.

The palate is formed by 2 shelf-like processes, developing from those surfaces of the maxillary processes, which are *inside* the primitive oral cavity. The 2 *palatal processes* first grow downward, along the sides of the developing tongue. By the middle or the end of the eighth week, the tongue muscles are capable of contractions and the tongue moves out of the way of the palatal processes. These are now released and flip up into a horizontal position, and their edges establish contact with each other, first in the front of the oral cavity and then gradually further backward (Figs. 7–16 and 7–17).

Fusion takes place between the touching edges of the palatal processes and the structure in the midline, formed by the combined medial nasal processes. Fusion involves a "glueing" together of the touching edges of these 3 structures. A cellular glue is produced by the epithelial cells covering the edges. Subsequently, these epithelial cells break down, so that the epithelial "seams" disappear and contact is established between the mesenchymal cores. The process of fusion is shown schematically in Figure 7–13 C, D.

Fusion of the palate occurs in a zipper-like fashion from the front to the back, from 8 weeks until 12 weeks, when the last part of the soft palate fuses. If fusion fails to occur, or if the epithelium fails to break down, or if either occurs incompletely, a cleft palate may result. Cleft palate may be found isolated or associated with a cleft lip. It may be unilateral or bilateral (Fig. 7–18).

DEVELOPMENT OF THE TONGUE. During the development of the external face, from the fourth through the sixth weeks, the tongue forms from 5 independent swellings on the inside surfaces (pharyngeal surfaces) of the first through the fourth arches in the neck region.

The grooves between these individual swellings of the tongue are eliminated in a manner similar to the groove elimination of the external face (Fig. 7–19).

In the fully developed tongue, the body of the tongue is formed by contributions from arches 1 and 2. The root or base of the tongue is formed by contributions from arches 3 and 4.

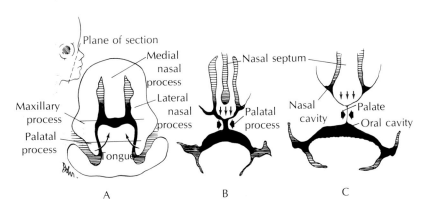

Fig. 7–16. *The development of the definitive palate in the seventh and eighth weeks of human embryonic development is shown in oblique, nearly vertical sections through the facial region (at the level indicated in the diagram at the far left), at 3 consecutive stages. Initially, the 2 palatal processes grow downward, alongside the tongue, growing out vertically from the inside surfaces of the maxillary processes, A. Subsequently, the tongue moves out of the way and the palatal processes flip up into a horizontal position (arrows). The 3 epithelially lined processes (combined medial nasal processes and 2 palatal processes) then are fused, B and C, in the manner shown in Figure 7–13 C and D.*

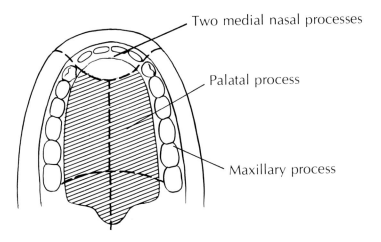

Two medial nasal processes

Palatal process

Maxillary process

Fig. 7–18.   A diagram of the hard and soft palates, as they appear viewed from below. The area of the front teeth corresponds with the primitive palate, formed largely by the 2 medial nasal processes. The shaded part of the palate (part of the hard palate in front, and the soft palate in the back) is formed by the 2 palatal processes, which come together and fuse in the midline. Clefts are possible at the fusion lines between the medial nasal processes and the palatal processes and in the midline between the 2 palatal processes.

Fig. 7–17.   A, Vertical section through the facial region of a 7-week-old human embryo. The 2 darkly staining eyes are included in the section. The tongue (T) and the palatal processes (PP), growing downward vertically along its sides, are clearly visible. LJ = lower jaw complex. Original magnification × 5. B, Oblique, nearly vertical section through the facial region of an 8.5-week-old human fetus. The palatal processes have moved up and have become fused with each other and with the nasal septum in a horizontal position. Some epithelial remnants (arrows) are still present in the midline seam between the palatal processes. Original magnification × 5.

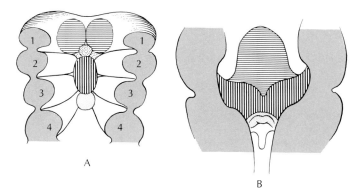

A

B

Fig. 7–19. Several, originally independent swellings, on the inside surfaces of the first through fourth arches in the embryo's neck region, participate in the formation of the tongue. The swellings are shown in a 3-dimensional view (from the inside) of the 4 arches in a 4-week-old embryo, A. At a somewhat later stage, B, the individual arches are no longer recognizable, and the grooves between the adjacent swellings have been eliminated. Some swellings have overgrown others, and a recognizable tongue is formed. Corresponding parts in the 2 diagrams are shaded identically.

SELECTED READING LIST

Johnston, M.C., Bhakdinarouk, A., and Reid, Y.C.: An expanded role of the neural crest in oral and pharyngeal development. In *Fourth Symposium on Oral Sensation and Perception. Development in the Fetus and Infant.* Edited by J.F. Bosma. Bethesda, MD, DHEW Publication No (NIH) 75-546, 1973.

Kraus, B.S., Kitamura, H., and Latham, R.A.: *Atlas of Developmental Anatomy of the Face. With Special Reference to Normal and Cleft Lip and Palate.* New York, Harper & Row, 1966.

Moore, K.L.: *The Developing Human. Clinically Oriented Embryology.* 2nd Ed. Philadelphia, W.B. Saunders Co., 1977.

Nishimura, H., Semba, R., Tanimura, T., and Tanaka, O.: Prenatal development of the human with special reference to craniofacial structures: an atlas. Bethesda, MD, DHEW Publication No (NIH) 77-946, 1977.

Noden, D.M.: The migratory behavior of neural crest cells. In *Fourth Symposium on Oral Sensation and Perception. Development in the Fetus and Infant.* Edited by J.F. Bosma. Bethesda, MD, DHEW Publication No (NIH) 75-546, 1973.

Sperber, G.H.: *Craniofacial Embryology.* 2nd Ed. Dental Practitioners Handbook #15. Bristol, John Wright and Sons, 1976.

Tuchmann-Duplessis, H., David, G., and Haegel, P.: *Illustrated Human Embryology. Vol. I. Embryogenesis.* New York, Springer Verlag, 1972.

DENTAL AND PERIODONTAL TISSUES

Chapter 8

INTRODUCTION TO PART II

In the second part of this book, Chapters 9 through 14, we will introduce the tissues of the tooth: enamel, dentin, pulp and cementum, and the tissues surrounding the tooth: alveolar bone, periodontal ligament and dentogingival junction.

When inspecting your own teeth in front of a mirror, try again to identify incisors, canines, premolars and molars. That part of a tooth which is visible inside the oral cavity is called the *crown* or, more precisely, the *clinical crown* of the tooth.

Another part of the tooth, which cannot be seen during inspection, is the *clinical root.* This is covered with gingiva and bone. Clinical roots may be seen in x-rays only.

The clinical crowns are shorter in young people than in older people because, with age, some of the bone is lost and the gingiva recedes, exposing more of the tooth to the oral cavity.

The tooth is a *complex* structure, consisting of 4 different "dental tissues": enamel, dentin, pulp and cementum.

The pulp is located in the center of a tooth, and it is surrounded by a dentin shell. Dentin is found in both the (anatomical) crown and the root of the tooth. The dentin in the crown is covered by an enamel cap; the dentin in the root is covered with cementum. The borderline between enamel and cementum is located at the neck or *cervix* of the tooth. This is also the borderline between *anatomical root* and *crown* (Fig. 8–1).

The part of the tooth that is covered with enamel is the anatomical crown; the part covered with cementum is the anatomical root. Notice that anatomical crown and root are not necessarily identical with clinical crown and root.

Between the gingiva and the surface of the tooth, a special junction, the *dentogingival junction,* is present. In young individuals, this junction is located entirely on the enamel surface. With age and the recession of the gingival tissues, the junction moves slowly onto the cementum, exposing more of the height of the tooth.

Thus, in young individuals, the clinical crown (the part of the tooth that is exposed) is *shorter* than the anatomical crown (the part

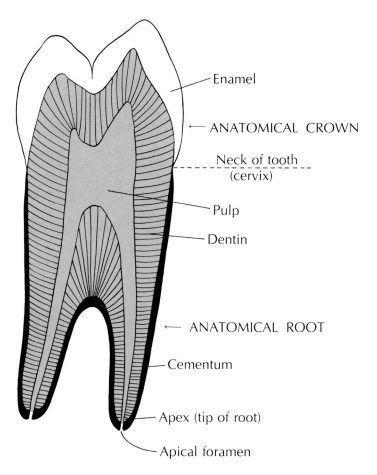

Enamel

ANATOMICAL CROWN

Neck of tooth
(cervix)

Pulp

Dentin

ANATOMICAL ROOT

Cementum

Apex (tip of root)

Apical foramen

Fig. 8–1. Diagram of a section through the entire length of a human tooth (premolar). The anatomical crown is the part of the tooth that is covered with enamel. The anatomical root is that part of the tooth that is covered with cementum. The neck (cervix) of the tooth is found where the anatomical crown meets the anatomical root. Both anatomical crown and root have a central core of dental pulp (uncalcified, loose connective tissue), surrounded by a shell of dentin. The tip of a dental root is the apex. At the apex an apical foramen gives access to the pulp chamber.

of the tooth that is covered with enamel). With recession of the gingiva, the clinical crown becomes taller, first reaching the same height as the anatomical crown, and subsequently becoming taller than the anatomical crown (Fig. 8–2).

Enamel is a calcified tissue that is deposited by epithelial (ectodermal) cells. After enamel has been formed, these epithelial cells are lost and enamel becomes a tissue without cells. This means that enamel, once formed, changes little. It does not increase in

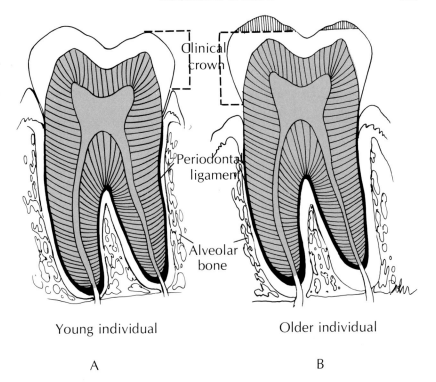

Young individual   Older individual

A   B

Fig. 8–2. Diagrams of sections of human molar teeth and the surrounding tissues in a young individual, A, and in a much older individual, B. Each tooth is suspended in a socket of alveolar bone, to which it is attached by means of a periodontal ligament. A, The height of the clinical crown (the exposed part of the tooth) is shorter than the height of the anatomical crown, since the latter is still partially covered with gingival tissues (free and attached gingiva). B, The gingival tissues and the upper rim of the alveolar bone socket have receded in the direction of the apices. This exposes all of the anatomical crown and even a small part of the anatomical root. The entire exposed part of the tooth is the clinical crown, which at this stage is of greater height than the anatomical crown. Other age changes include: wear of the enamel cap (and sometimes some dentin as well), increased thickness of dentin and thus a decreased size of the pulp, and a thicker layer of cementum, especially near the apices.

thickness and has no healing ability to repair damages of caries and wear.

Dentin and cementum are both *calcified connective tissues.* Dentin is capable of continued appositional growth in an inward direction. This does not affect the external dimensions of a tooth, but it does encroach upon the centrally located pulp tissue. With age, the dentin layer becomes thicker and the pulp chamber becomes correspondingly smaller.

Cementum is also capable of continued appositional growth in an outward direction. Thus, with age, the cementum layer becomes thicker, especially near the tip, or *apex*, of the root.

Pulp is an uncalcified, *loose connective tissue*. It contains the blood vessels and nerves necessary for the vitality of the tooth. The pulp is enclosed almost entirely by dentin. Only at the apex, through the *apical foramen*, is the pulp in contact with other connective tissues.

The borderline between dentin and enamel in the anatomical crown is called the *dentino-enamel junction*. The borderline between dentin and cementum in the anatomical root is called the *dentino-cementum junction*. The borderline between cementum and enamel at the cervix of the tooth is called the *cemento-enamel junction*.

We distinguish 3 "periodontal tissues": dentogingival junction (epithelium), alveolar bone and periodontal ligament (connective tissue).

The anatomical root of a tooth is suspended in an individual bone socket or *alveolus*. The root is attached to this socket by means of a *dense connective tissue*, consisting primarily of highly organized, tendon-like collagen fiber bundles. This is the *periodontal ligament*. The periodontal ligament forms a specialized *joint* between the tooth and the alveolar bone, somewhat comparable to a suture.

In the following chapters, we will describe each of these dental and periodontal tissues in greater detail.

Chapter 9

TOOTH DEVELOPMENT AND ERUPTION

Tooth development takes place over a long period of time. It begins in the seventh week of embryonic life (primary dentition), and it continues well into the late teenage years (third molar of the secondary dentition).

The following occurs during this period: (1) a *primary* dentition (milk dentition, deciduous dentition), consisting of 20 teeth, develops, erupts, functions and is shed; and (2) a *secondary* dentition (permanent dentition), consisting of 32 teeth, develops, erupts (replacing in part the teeth of the primary dentition) and becomes functional.

From a clinical point of view, there are 2 important facts that require an understanding of tooth development:

1. Young children and teenagers who are seen in the dental office have teeth that are in several different stages of development. Clinically visible teeth may be part of a *mixed* dentition (teeth of both primary and secondary dentitions are functional). Other teeth are not visible, but are still in the process of developing in the underlying tissues of the jaw. You should be prepared to recognize such teeth clinically as well as radiographically. From the standpoint of prevention, if developing teeth are present in the jaw, nutritional counseling and the restricted use of certain drugs, such as tetracyclines (see Chap. 10), are desirable to prevent developmental anomalies of the developing teeth.

2. You should also be aware that the presence of many developing teeth leaves little space for bone tissue in a child's jaw, and can result in a weakening of the jaw structure, making it more susceptible to trauma, i.e., fractures (Fig. 9–1).

At the end of this chapter, timetables for the emergence of the various teeth into the oral cavity, as well as reviews of the various developmental stages of the 2 dentitions, may be found. But first we will discuss the principal events in the process of tooth development.

Fig. 9–1. Skulls of a 4½-year-old child, A, *and a 9-year-old child,* B. *The outer bone layers of upper and lower jaws have been removed to expose the teeth of the secondary dentition, which have not yet erupted and become functional.* A, *Only the teeth of the primary dentition are functional. The upper and lower jaws are filled with developing teeth of the secondary dentition, leaving little space for bone tissue.* B, *The incisors and the first molars of the secondary dentition have become functional. Secondary canines, premolars and second molars are still developing inside the jaws, the canines and premolars beneath the roots of their primary predecessors.*

TOOTH DEVELOPMENT

As noted in Chapter 8, a tooth is a complex structure, consisting of 4 tissues: 3 *calcified* tissues (enamel, dentin and cementum) and 1 *noncalcified* tissue (dental pulp).

Of these 4 tissues, dentin, cementum and pulp are classified as connective tissues, while enamel may be classified as a product of epithelial cells. Developmentally, the tooth is the product of 2 *basic* tissues: embryonic connective tissue (the jaw mesenchyme, derived from neural crest) and (2) epithelial tissue (oral epithelium, derived from ectoderm).

The jaw mesenchyme and the oral epithelium interact complexly with each other during the formation of the tooth. The epithelium itself is unable to form enamel unless the jaw mesenchyme is present, and conversely, the mesenchyme cannot form dentin, pulp or cementum unless the oral epithelium, or at least some epithelial product, is present.

In tooth development 2 principal events must occur: (1) the establishment of the particular tooth *shapes* by a process called *morphodifferentiation;* and (2) the *differentiation* of special groups of cells into dentin-forming cells *(odontoblasts),* enamel-forming

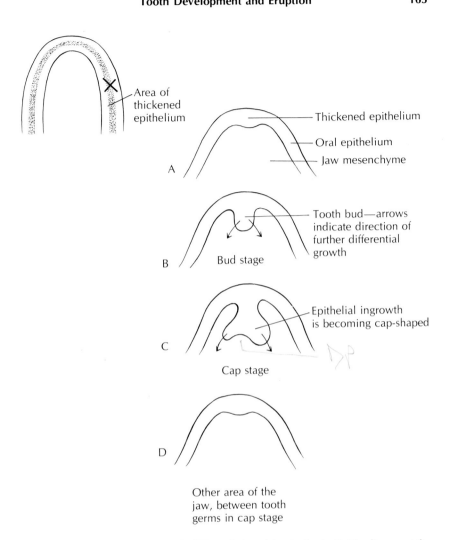

Fig. 9–2. Early stages in the morphodifferentiation of developing teeth. The diagram at the left top shows the oral surface of a jaw. A horseshoe-shaped thickening of oral epithelium (stippled) is formed along the surface of the jaw. The epithelium grows into the underlying mesenchyme. x indicates the plane of section through the jaw, shown in diagrams A through C. A, The first development of thickened epithelium. At the slightly later stage, B, bud-like thickenings have formed in specific areas, corresponding with the locations of future teeth. Differential growth of the epithelium in each of these buds leads to the formation of epithelial caps in the next phase of development, C. The arrows indicate the preferential directions of epithelial growth, leading to the formation of the cap-shape. The caps remain attached for a while to the oral epithelium by an epithelial sheet (shown as a strand in cross section): the dental lamina. D, Section through the jaw (at the same phase of development as shown in C) in an area between the locations of developing teeth. Here no further development takes place beyond the stage of thickened epithelium.

cells *(ameloblasts)*, cementum-forming cells *(cementoblasts)* and pulp-forming cells *(fibroblasts)*, by a process called *cytodifferentiation*.

Morphodifferentiation

The main stages of morphodifferentiation, for both primary and secondary tooth development, are bud stage, cap stage and bell stage (Fig. 9–2).

The oral epithelium, growing into the underlying mesenchyme of the jaw, is responsible for the shaping of the tooth. This process

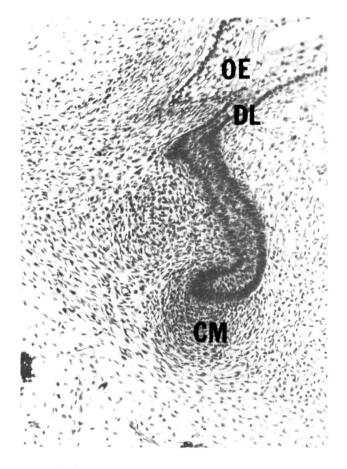

Fig. 9–3. Tooth development in early cap stage. The development from bud to cap stage is frequently uneven. In this case one half of the epithelial cap is further along in development than the other half. OE = oral epithelium; DL = dental lamina; CM = condensed mesenchyme. Original magnification × 20.

begins when the oral epithelium starts to thicken locally and extends on both sides, forming a horseshoe shape that follows the curve of the future dental arches. The thickened oral epithelium begins to proliferate into the underlying mesenchyme.

As the result of the different rates of growth in the various parts of this proliferating epithelium, the ingrowth locally becomes thickened into *buds (bud stage)*. Each epithelial bud is associated with a sphere of *condensed mesenchyme* (Fig. 9–3).

These buds form only in areas where teeth will develop. There are, therefore, 10 buds in the upper jaw and 10 in the lower jaw, which go on to form the teeth of the primary dentition. Later 16

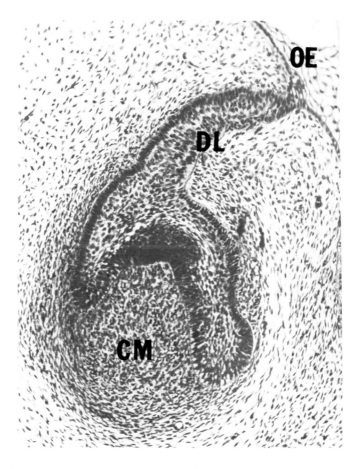

Fig. 9–4. Tooth development in the cap stage. A clear cap-shape has been established by the ingrowing epithelium. Spaces have begun to develop between the epithelial cells in the center of the cap. OE = oral epithelium; DL = dental lamina; CM = condensed mesenchyme. Original magnification × 20.

buds in the upper jaw and 16 in the lower jaw initiate the development of the teeth of the secondary dentition. Between the buds, the epithelium does not proliferate further downward and remains just a thickened band.

Differential growth of parts of the buds changes the shapes of these epithelial structures into *caps (cap stage)*. In this stage the future shape of the tooth becomes evident. With continued growth

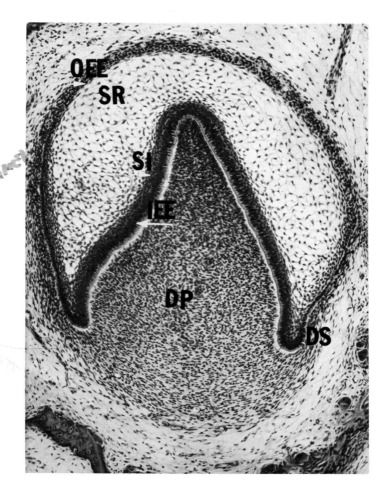

Fig. 9–5. Tooth development in the early bell stage. There is a clear differentiation in the epithelial enamel organ between the cells of the outer enamel epithelium (OEE), stellate reticulum (SR), stratum intermedium (SI) and inner enamel epithelium (IEE). The condensed mesenchyme inside the enamel organ is the dental papilla (DP). The condensed mesenchyme around the enamel organ is the dental sac (DS). Around the tooth germ, a much-less-condensed mesenchyme is visible and some of the developing bone of the jaw (darkly staining). No dental lamina is visible since this section is somewhat off-center through the enamel organ. Original magnification × 20.

and differentiation the caps become highly specialized epithelial organs: *enamel organs*. These enamel organs reach full morphodifferentiation in the next stage, the *bell stage* (Figs. 9–4 and 9–5).

The bell stage is the final stage of morphodifferentiation. During this stage the first cytodifferentiation occurs within the enamel organ itself, resulting in the establishment of 4 distinct epithelial layers: outer enamel epithelium, stellate reticulum, stratum intermedium and inner enamel epithelium (Fig. 9–6).

Let us have a closer look at a developing tooth in the bell stage. A developing tooth, or *tooth germ,* consists of 2 components: the *epithelial* and the *mesenchymal.*

Fig. 9–6. Two tooth germs (incisors of the primary dentition) in the final bell stage of development. At the end of the bell stage, and during the earliest deposition of the hard dental tissues, the shaping process of the dentino-enamel junction (in the anatomical crown) by the inner enamel epithelium (IEE) is nearly completed. The stellate reticulum (SR) is extensive. A very thin layer of dentin has been deposited near the incisal edges. The tooth germ of the incisor at the left is somewhat tilted. This results in a sectioned image, resembling the section through the side of a bowl. Original magnification × 6.

The *epithelial component* (the enamel organ), in the bell stage, undergoes cytodifferentiation into the 4 distinct layers already outlined. The innermost layer, the inner enamel epithelium, which lines the concave inner surface of the enamel organ, will be responsible for the formation of enamel. The stratum intermedium and the stellate reticulum will support and assist the inner enamel epithelium in this future function.

The *mesenchymal* is further subdivided into the *dental papilla* and the *dental sac*. The *dental papilla* is condensed mesenchyme located in the concavity of the enamel organ. The peripheral cells will form dentin, while the central part of the dental papilla will further develop into the dental pulp. The *dental sac* (dental follicle) is condensed mesenchyme that surrounds the convex surface of the

Fig. 9–7. Histologic section through the cervical loop of an enamel organ in the bell stage. At this loop, inner and outer enamel epithelia meet. Two mitotic figures are visible (asterisks), evidence that this part of the enamel organ is characterized by very active growth. Original magnification × 500.

enamel organ. It supplies the cells that will form cementum, the periodontal ligament and part of the alveolar bone socket of the tooth.

The epithelial strand, which still connects the enamel organ with the oral epithelium, is the *dental lamina*. It has no further role once tooth development has progressed this far, and it will fall apart. However, some epithelial cells of the dental lamina may stay behind as strands or as clumps. These cell remnants may undergo further mitoses and occasionally even some central keratinization. If that occurs, they may enlarge and become visible as little white bumps beneath the oral mucosa of a baby. Usually no complications result, and these structures are lost during the process of tooth eruption, when the tooth emerges through the oral epithelium into the oral cavity.

Before discussing *cytodifferentiation,* we should make 2 important points:

1. *Overlap* of morphodifferentiation and cytodifferentiation periods. You may have noticed in Figures 9–5 and 9–6, depicting tooth development, that the shaping of a tooth is a gradual process. The first part of a tooth to be shaped is the part that is nearest to the oral epithelium: the future cusps of a molar or the incisal edge of an incisor. The rest of the crown is gradually further shaped in an

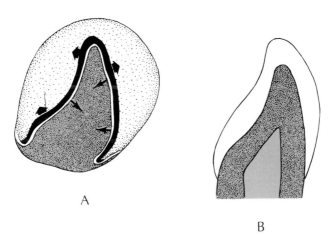

A

B

Fig. 9–8.   Diagrams showing a tooth germ in the bell stage, A, and the anatomical crown of a fully formed tooth, B. The dentino-enamel junction is shaped by the inner enamel epithelium (dark band in A). During the deposition stage, the inner enamel epithelial cells move backward (large arrows) while depositing enamel matrix, and the mesenchymal cells of the dental papilla move backward (small arrows) while depositing dentin. Thus, the location of the inner enamel epithelium in the bell stage is preserved as the interface between enamel and dentin (the dentino-enamel junction) in the fully formed tooth. Enamel: blank in B; dentin: stippled in B.

occlusocervical direction, and only when the shape of the crown is established fully will the root be shaped.

The structure responsible for this continued shaping process is the *cervical loop* (Fig. 9–7). The cervical loop is the cervical-most rim of the enamel organ, where outer and inner enamel epithelia meet. Mitoses of the epithelial cells in this rim are responsible for the continued growth of the cervical loop, thereby shaping first the rest of the crown and later the root.

This process of *morpho*differentiation takes place while in the occluso-incisal region *cyto*differentiation is well advanced. Therefore the oldest part of the tooth, with respect to both morphodifferentiation and cytodifferentiation, is its incisal edge or cusp; the youngest part of a tooth is the tip, or apex, of its root.

2. The *precise part* of the future tooth, which is shaped by the differential growth of the epithelial enamel organ. On the preceding pages we have indicated that the inner enamel epithelium establishes the shape of a tooth. The exact part of the tooth to be shaped by the epithelium is the *borderline* between dentin and enamel, the dentino-enamel junction. This borderline reflects the exact position of the borderline between dental papilla and inner enamel epithelium at the conclusion of the morphodifferentiation process and at the beginning of the cytodifferentiation process (Fig. 9–8).

Cytodifferentiation

Cytodifferentiation is the result of a series of *cellular* interactions between epithelial and mesenchymal components of the tooth germs.

As we stated before, in order for a tooth to develop, the presence of both epithelial and mesenchymal components is essential. The reason for this is that these 2 tissues continuously communicate with each other, *both* during morphodifferentiation *and* during cytodifferentiation. Alternate messages move across the *basal lamina,* the boundary between epithelium and mesenchyme.

1. The first communication comes from the mesenchyme in the early stages of morphodifferentiation. This message, on reaching the oral epithelium, instructs the epithelium to grow downward into the mesenchyme and shape the tooth.

It is now clear that the mesenchyme is the important determinant both for the *initiation* of tooth development and for the specific *type* of tooth (incisor vs. molar for instance). The precise nature of the message is not known at this time. It is possible that the mesenchymal cells produce a substance that serves as a message for the initiation of tooth development (perhaps a protein). If the message in fact consists of such a substance, it must diffuse, through the basal lamina, from the mesenchyme to the epithelial cells and stimulate the latter to undergo the greater numbers of mitoses that are necessary for *morphodifferentiation.*

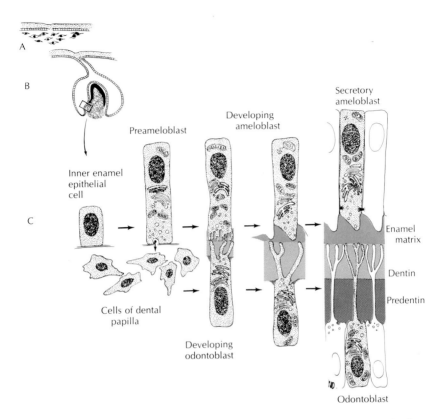

A

B

Secretory
ameloblast

Developing
ameloblast

Preameloblast

Inner enamel
epithelial
cell

C

Enamel
matrix

Dentin

Predentin

Cells of dental
papilla

Developing
odontoblast

Odontoblast

*Fig. 9–9.   Sequence of cell interactions and cytodifferentiations during tooth develop-
ment. A, The initiation of tooth development. A message crosses the basal lamina from
mesenchyme to epithelium. The epithelium responds by downgrowth and differentiation
into an enamel organ. B, The outline of an enamel organ is shown. The dental papilla is
stippled. A dark strip of dentin is present in the incisal region. A small area is shown in
greater detail in C. While all stages of cytodifferentiation, illustrated in C, can be found
simultaneously in a single tooth germ at this stage of development, it should be remembered
that each epithelial cell and each odontoblast will undergo all these stages of development
sequentially. Initially, the inner enamel epithelial cell becomes a taller preameloblast. This
preameloblast produces a substance that is transmitted through the basal lamina (arrow)
and reaches some of the mesenchymal cells of the dental papilla. These cells now develop
into tall odontoblasts and begin to synthesize predentin. The basal lamina disappears and
the cell processes of the developing odontoblast come in close contact with the cell
processes of the preameloblast. Subsequently, the preameloblast differentiates into an
ameloblast and starts producing enamel matrix. Because the odontoblast starts its
productive activities some time before the ameloblast, the dentin layer in any location in a
developing tooth is thicker than the corresponding layer of enamel matrix.*

Fig. 9–10.   Stages of odontoblast and ameloblast differentiation, seen in histologic section.
A, Inner enamel epithelial cells face the undifferentiated mesenchymal cells of the dental
papilla. A basement membrane intervenes between the 2. B, Elongation of inner enamel
epithelial cells into preameloblasts. Stellate reticulum and stratum intermedium are visible.
C, Alignment of the mesenchymal cells along the basal lamina (starting at the level of the
asterisk). Differentiation of the odontoblasts begins.

Fig. 9–10. (Cont'd). D, *First dentin deposition by the newly differentiated odontoblasts. The preameloblasts begin to differentiate further.* E, *Ameloblasts, with Tomes' processes, are engaged in enamel matrix deposition. Dentin and predentin are visible. Key to abbreviations: IEE = inner enamel epithelium; SI = stratum intermedium; SR = stellate reticulum; M = mesenchymal cells; PA = preameloblasts; A = ameloblasts; O = Odontoblasts; PD = predentin; D = dentin; EM = enamel matrix; TP = Tomes' processes. Original magnification × 125.*

2. Cytodifferentiation of Odontoblasts. The second message is given by the cells of the inner enamel epithelium to the mesenchymal cells in the periphery of the dental papilla. Again, it should be remembered that this is a *sequential* process. Cytodifferentiation (Figs. 9–9 and 9–10) begins occlusally or incisally and moves in a gradual, wave-like fashion toward the cervix of the tooth. In order to give the message to the mesenchymal cells, the cells of the inner enamel epithelium must have completed the process of morphodifferentiation at their level in the tooth. This means that the inner enamel epithelial cells have stopped dividing. They grow taller and more columnar, and their nuclei move from the central position to that part of the cell which faces away from the basal lamina. In this way a *polarity* is established in the inner enamel epithelial cells.

All these changes are the result of the development of large amounts of protein-synthesizing organelles in these cells. The elongated epithelial cells are now called *pre-ameloblasts,* and the first product they synthesize is secreted into the basal lamina. We do not yet know what kind of product this is: a simple protein, or a protein associated with carbohydrate chains. However, we do know that this product contains a message for the peripheral cells of the dental papilla, whose cell processes touch the basal lamina, which contains this product.

The message, once received by the mesenchymal cells, permits these cells to undergo differentiation. Once differentiated, these *odontoblasts* line up along the basal lamina. The cytodifferentiation of the odontoblasts involves the formation of large amounts of organelles, which will eventually synthesize the components of the fibrous matrix and the ground substance of dentin.

The odontoblasts elongate during their differentiation, and their nuclei move away from the basal lamina (polarization). Differentiated odontoblasts are no longer able to undergo mitosis.

3. *Cytodifferentiation of Ameloblasts.* As soon as the odontoblasts have differentiated and have begun to produce dentin matrix, another communication is necessary for the cytodifferentiation of the ameloblasts (Figs. 9–9 and 9–10). Once again, it is the turn of the mesenchyme, now the differentiated odontoblasts, to give the message to the epithelium, now the pre-ameloblasts. For this final message the basal lamina between the 2 cell types has to break down. Across the broken-down basal lamina, the odontoblasts and pre-ameloblasts push cell extensions toward each other. These extensions make *temporary contacts,* and it is now felt that, during this brief period of contact, the odontoblasts give a message to the pre-ameloblasts, permitting the latter to become *ameloblasts* and begin enamel matrix production.

We should emphasize here that each of the aforementioned interactions between epithelial and mesenchymal cells is a prerequisite for the further development of the tooth. If the pre-ameloblasts fail to give a message to the odontoblasts, the next interaction, the communication between odontoblasts and pre-ameloblasts (for the cytodifferentiation of the ameloblasts), cannot occur either.

Dentin and Enamel Formation

There are some similarities between the processes of enamel and dentin formation, and some differences.

SIMILARITIES. Both odontoblasts and ameloblasts are polarized cells. With their secretory sides they face the basal lamina, while the nuclei are located in the opposite ends of the cells. During dentin and enamel production, the odontoblasts and the ameloblasts both move away from their original positions next to the basal lamina, leaving their products behind. Since ameloblasts and odontoblasts are located on opposite sides of the basal lamina, they move away from this structure, the future dentino-enamel junction, in *opposite directions* (Fig. 9–11).

DIFFERENCES. The *odontoblasts* produce a *connective tissue* product that resembles bone. The product consists of a fibrous

Fig. 9–11.   Histologic section of a developing tooth at the time of enamel and dentin formation. The arrows indicate the directions in which ameloblasts (A) and odontoblasts (O) move, while depositing their products. The darkest staining layer is enamel matrix; the somewhat lighter staining tissue next to it is the dentin. At the bottom right of this picture, the odontoblasts are just differentiating. Original magnification × 50.

matrix, with predominantly collagen fibers, and a carbohydrate-rich ground substance, which binds some water. The *ameloblasts,* on the other hand, are epithelial cells, and they produce a rather distinct and unique *epithelial product.* The enamel matrix is known to consist of proteins and proteins bound to carbohydrates, but the precise nature of these substances is as yet unclear.

At some distance from the receding odontoblasts, the *dentin matrix* begins to undergo calcification. Hydroxyapatite salts are deposited in this matrix. Between the odontoblasts and the calcification front, a strip of uncalcified *predentin* (like the osteoid seam in bone) is present (Fig. 9–12).

The *enamel matrix,* produced by the ameloblasts, contains a small amount of hydroxyapatite, almost from the moment it is laid down; therefore, *no* wide strip of uncalcified enamel matrix is present. The small crystals of hydroxyapatite salt, *hydroxyapatite crystallites,* are delicate, and a relatively large amount of enamel matrix is found between them. Enamel undergoes, at a somewhat later time, an unusual process called *maturation.* During this process, it becomes the most heavily calcified tissue of the body. The maturation consists of an *enlargement* of the hydroxyapatite crystallites, already present in the enamel matrix. This enlargement occurs at the expense of the matrix, which *in part* is broken down and *removed* by the same ameloblasts that originally deposited this matrix. The ameloblasts have, therefore, *successively* a synthetic stage and a digestive stage (with lysosomal activities) (Figs. 9–13 and 9–14).

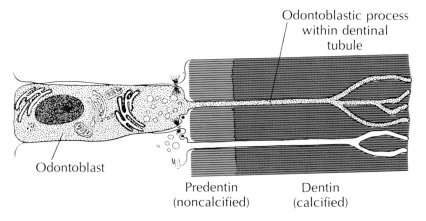

Odontoblastic process
within dentinal
tubule

Odontoblast

Predentin
(noncalcified)

Dentin
(calcified)

Fig. 9–12. Diagram of an odontoblast, actively engaged in dentin formation. The various organelles associated with protein synthesis are found in the odontoblastic cell body. Each odontoblast leaves an odontoblastic process behind inside a dentinal tubule. The seam of newly formed dentin is noncalcified predentin. It undergoes calcification and becomes dentin at a short distance from the retreating odontoblasts.

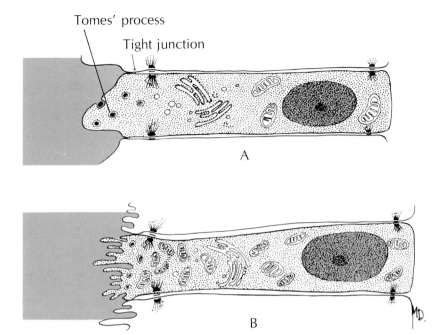

Tomes' process

Tight junction

A

B

Fig. 9–13.   The appearance of an ameloblast during its synthetic (secretory) stage, A, and during its digestive (back resorptive) stage, B, which occurs later. A, The ameloblast has the typical organelles, associated with synthetic activities. Secretory granules are released from a typical, somewhat conical cell extension: the Tomes' process. This process is present only during the secretory stage. During certain phases of the digestive stage, B, the ameloblast has the typical organelles associated with digestive activities, as well as a ruffled border, facing the enamel matrix.

When the *odontoblasts* move backward and produce dentin matrix, they do not ordinarily become enclosed in this matrix (unlike the osteoblasts, which may become osteocytes). However, each odontoblast leaves one long, cytoplasmic cell extension, an *odontoblastic process,* behind in the dentin matrix. This dentin matrix encloses the odontoblastic processes in individual tubes or *dentinal tubules.* Throughout the life of the tooth, the odontoblasts and their processes remain a vital part of the dentin tissue that they produced.

The *ameloblasts,* on the other hand, are lost when the tooth emerges into the oral cavity during eruption. Since no cells are associated with mature enamel, strictly speaking, enamel is not a true tissue, although it is usually called a tissue. It is a secretion product, incapable of repair once it is formed. During the period of enamel matrix production, the ameloblasts have a shovel-shaped

cytoplasmic extension with a wide base and a thin outer edge at their secretory surface. As we shall see later, this extension (Tomes' process) is responsible for the particular pattern in which enamel matrix is laid down.

Both dentin and enamel formation begin at the dentino-enamel junction of the cusps or incisal edges of the various teeth. Since the odontoblasts undergo cytodifferentiation somewhat earlier than the ameloblasts in the corresponding locations, dentin formation is somewhat further advanced cervically than enamel formation at any given time during dental crown development.

In the absence of serious complications, the production of dentin and of enamel is an orderly process. The cellular sheets, formed by the layer of odontoblasts and the layer of ameloblasts, behave as 2 organic units. This is possible because of the presence of gap junctions and tight junctions, which allow odontoblasts to communicate freely with neighboring odontoblasts and ameloblasts to communicate similarly with neighboring ameloblasts.

Depending on their location in a particular tooth, odontoblasts and ameloblasts produce, on the average, about 4 μm of both dentin and enamel daily.

Root Development

Root development begins when the enamel organ has shaped the crown completely and when the developing tooth has started its eruptive movement.

MORPHODIFFERENTIATION. The root is shaped by further epithelial downgrowth. Remember that during the morphodifferentiation of the crown, the occlusal/incisal surfaces are shaped first, and that continued growth of the cervical loop is responsible for further shaping of the rest of the crown. When the

Fig. 9–14. Decalcified histologic section, A, ground section, B, and an x-ray of a ground section, C, of the same primary tooth and its secondary successor. Notice that the enamel of the primary tooth is absent in the decalcified section, present in the ground section and very radiopaque (white) in the x-ray. This reflects the fact that mature enamel is highly calcified, with so little enamel matrix that the matrix disintegrates during decalcification. In the developing tooth, the most recently deposited enamel matrix (near the cervix) is still present in the decalcified section, but near the incisal edge, the older enamel is maturing (acquiring more mineral and losing matrix components). The x-ray shows also that more mineral is present near the incisal edge and along the dentino-enamel junction than in the remainder of the developing enamel. Original magnification A and B, × 2. C, × 4. (Courtesy the late Dr. E. Applebaum.)

entire crown is shaped, and cytodifferentiation has led to the
development of the 4 layers of the enamel organ (inner and outer
enamel epithelia, stratum intermedium and stellate reticulum), the
outer and inner enamel epithelia, which meet at the cervical loop,
begin to proliferate further apically. These 2 layers of epithelium
form the epithelial root sheath (Hertwig's sheath). Its function is the
shaping of the root or roots and the induction of the odontoblasts, to
deposit the dentin of the roots.

As is the case in the crown, the epithelial root sheath does *not*

Fig. 9–15. *During early morphodifferentiation of a dental root, an epithelial root sheath*
(arrow) grows apically, shaping the future dentino-cementum junction by inducing the
odontoblasts, which will form the root dentin. At the level of the asterisk, cells from the
dental sac have moved between the remnants of the root sheath and the surface of the
dentin, where they will differentiate into cementoblasts. Original magnification ×40.

shape the outer surface of the root, but rather <u>the dentinocementum junction</u>. The epithelial root sheath proliferates apically at approximately the same rate at which the developing tooth is erupting. As a result, the growing tip of the root remains in about the same position within the jaw (Figs. 9–15, 9–16 and 9–17).

The inner enamel epithelium of the root sheath faces the dental papilla, but is separated from it by the basal lamina. The outer enamel epithelium faces the dental sac, but is separated from it by a basal lamina which is continuous with the basal lamina between dental papilla and inner enamel epithelium.

CYTODIFFERENTIATION OF ODONTOBLASTS. The inner enamel epithelium of the root sheath induces the peripheral cells of the dental papilla to differentiate into odontoblasts. This

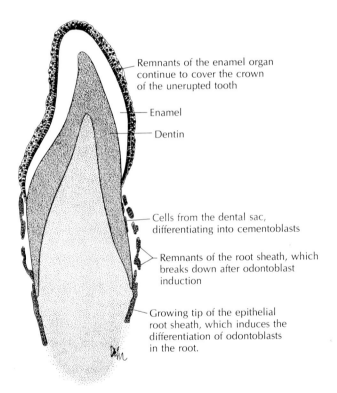

Remnants of the enamel organ
continue to cover the crown
of the unerupted tooth

Enamel

Dentin

Cells from the dental sac,
differentiating into cementoblasts

Remnants of the root sheath, which
breaks down after odontoblast
induction

Growing tip of the epithelial
root sheath, which induces the
differentiation of odontoblasts
in the root.

Fig. 9–16. *Diagram of root development. The growing tip of the epithelial root sheath continues to proliferate apically, further shaping the dentino-cementum junction of the anatomical root. Once the first root dentin has been deposited, the root sheath breaks down. Between the epithelial remnants, cells of the dental sac move to the root dentin surface, where they will differentiate into cementoblasts. While all these stages can be seen in one developing tooth, they will all take place in sequence, at all points along the growing root from cervix to apex.*

Fig. 9–17.   Histologic section through the tip of an epithelial root sheath. This structure essentially consists of 2 layers of epithelial cells, one of which is continuous with the outer enamel epithelium, while the other is continuous with the inner enamel epithelium of the enamel organ. DP = dental papilla; DS = dental sac with cross sections through 2 blood vessels (BV). Original magnification × 400.

occurs in a manner that is similar to what takes place in the crown. When the odontoblasts are differentiated and begin to deposit dentin, the basal laminae on both sides of the epithelial root sheath break down, and the continuity of the root sheath itself is lost.

Unlike the ameloblasts in the enamel organ, the inner enamel epithelial cells of the root sheath do *not* undergo any further differentiation after they have induced the odontoblasts, and they do not seem to have any further function.

Before the root sheath breaks up, the epithelial cells may deposit a thin layer of proteins at the future dentinocementum junction, but this activity is negligible.

CYTODIFFERENTIATION OF CEMENTOBLASTS. The breakdown of the epithelial root sheath at the levels of the developing root at which dentin production has begun allows the undifferentiated mesenchymal cells of the dental sac to move toward the surface of the root dentin. In doing so, they push the epithelial remnants of the root sheath (cell rests of Malassez) further away from the root dentin. Some components of the recently deposited dentin matrix probably are responsible for the inductive message, which leads to the differentiation of the dental sac mesenchymal cells into *cementoblasts.* This involves the development of extensive rough, endoplasmic reticulum and Golgi systems.

The newly differentiated cementoblasts begin to deposit cementum on the dentin surface of the root. Cementum is first laid down as an uncalcified matrix (cementoid, similar to osteoid or predentin), which calcifies at some distance from the receding cementoblasts.

Little cementum is deposited before and during the emergence of the tooth in the oral cavity. Only after the tooth reaches functional occlusion is cementum deposited in substantial amounts. Some cementoblasts become enclosed by their product and are then called *cementocytes.* Cementoblasts and cementocytes remain associated with the tissue they produced, and cementum may be deposited throughout the functional life of the tooth (Fig. 9–18).

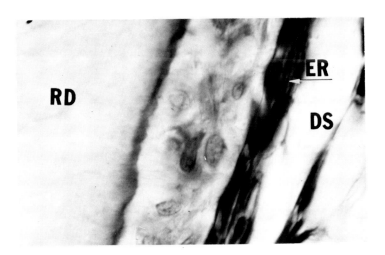

Fig. 9–18.   Histologic section through the future dentino-cementum junction of a developing tooth. RD = root dentin; DS = dental sac; ER = large epithelial remnant of the epithelial root sheath. Between the epithelial remnant and the root dentin, several dental sac cells have lined up along the dentin surface and have differentiated into cementoblasts. Early cementum deposition is taking place. Original magnification × 500.

Multirooted Teeth

In teeth with a single root, the epithelial root sheath simply grows apically, as an epithelial cylinder, from the cervical edge of the enamel organ. In teeth with 2 or 3 roots, the single cervical opening, bordered by the epithelial root sheath, must first be subdivided into 2 or 3 openings. This subdivision is done by the horizontal outgrowth of 2 or 3 epithelial flaps across the cervical opening. These flaps, consisting usually of 2 cell layers (inner and outer enamel epithelium, like the epithelial root sheath), meet in the center of the cervical opening, where they fuse. Now, from the edges of these newly formed, smaller openings, 2 or 3 cylindrical root sheaths grow apically, shaping 2 or 3 separate roots (Figs. 9–19 and 9–20).

Occasionally a tooth has a single root with 2 separate root canals in it. This situation is produced as follows: a single epithelial root sheath is present. A cross section through this root sheath reveals a gradual change from a circular to an oval outline, with central indentations (Fig. 9–21). The odontoblasts, differentiated within this

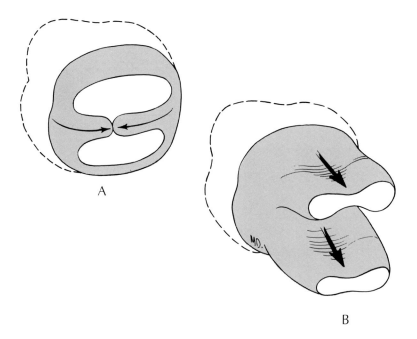

Fig. 9–19. Diagram of the development of a tooth with 2 separate roots. The broken outline reflects the anatomical crown region. The developing tooth is tilted on its side. **A,** *The outgrowth of 2 epithelial flaps* (arrows) *from the cervical loop, subdividing the single cervical opening into 2 separate openings. From the edges of both these openings, epithelial root sheaths grow apically,* **B** (arrows), *shaping 2 separate roots.*

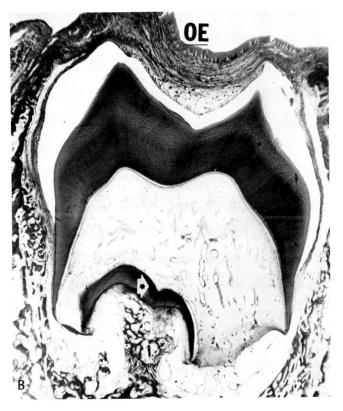

Fig. 9–20. A, Histologic section through a developing primary molar. The enamel organ is cut slightly off-center, so that the dentin and enamel formation, which is occurring in the cusp region, is not visible. A cross section through a small epithelial flap, which is growing across the cervical opening, is visible. This is the first stage in the root development of a multi-rooted tooth. Original magnification × 10. B, Histologic section through a developing primary molar, just before the tooth emerges into the oral cavity (OE = oral epithelium). This is a later stage in the development of 2 separate roots. The dentin, marked with an asterisk, has been produced by the odontoblasts, which were induced by the epithelial flaps subdividing the cervical opening. Original magnification × 2.

Fig. 9–21. The development of 2 separate root canals in a single root is shown in this diagram of a cross section through the root. When the root sheath has central indentations, subsequent even dentin production leads to a central obstruction and 2 separate root canals.

Fig. 9–22. Histologic section through the molar region in the lower jaw of a human fetus (second trimester of pregnancy). Developing primary canine (c), first and second primary molars (m_1 and m_2) and the enamel organ (cap stage) of the first molar of the secondary dentition (M_1) are visible. Most developing teeth still lie in a common bony groove, together with the major nerves and blood vessels of the lower jaw (arrow). No subdivision into individual bony crypts (and canal) has taken place as yet. Original magnification × 2. (Courtesy the late Dr. E. Applebaum.)

outline, produce dentin in a central direction, all at about the same rate. This leads to a rapid obliteration of the dental papilla in the central, indented region and to the establishment of 2 separate canals for the root pulp.

The Bony Crypts

During the early stages of dental development, intramembranous ossification is taking place in the upper and lower jaw regions. Soon, a delicate network of bone is formed, which partially surrounds the tooth germs. No bone forms in the spaces occupied by the enamel organs, their dental sacs, dental papillae and dental lamina or its remnants.

In these early stages, the individual tooth germs are all located in a common bony groove, whose outer edges curve gently inward, seemingly preventing the tooth germs from "falling out" of the bony groove. Subsequently, as growth continues and the teeth come to lie somewhat further apart, this common groove is subdivided into individual compartments or bony *crypts* (Fig. 9–22).

Innervation and Vascularization

Tooth development is an active metabolic process, requiring a great deal of energy. From the earliest stages of epithelial ingrowth, a large number of *capillaries* surrounds the spherical mass of condensed mesenchyme of the tooth germ.

In the cap and bell stages of tooth development, these capillaries invade the dental papilla and the dental sac. The future ameloblasts and odontoblasts initially both receive their nutrition from the capillaries in the dental papilla. When the odontoblasts have differentiated and are depositing dentin, the capillary network becomes even richer. Many capillaries lie in and immediately underneath the odontoblast layer.

However, the very deposition of dentin and enamel matrix now prevents the ameloblasts from receiving their nutrition from the dental papilla any longer. Suddenly, the rich capillary network in the dental sac, outside the outer enamel epithelium, becomes their source of nutrition and respiratory gases. These vessels come even closer to the ameloblasts because of the gradual *collapse* of the enamel organ, during the phase of enamel matrix deposition.

In addition to small capillaries, delicate nerve fibers are present in the dental papillae and the dental sacs as early as the cap and bell stages of dental development. The nerves in the dental papilla eventually grow toward the odontoblastic cell layer. But only *after* the odontoblasts have deposited a thick layer of dentin (about two-thirds of its future thickness) do the nerve fibers form terminals on the odontoblasts.

TOOTH MOVEMENTS AND TOOTH ERUPTION

Throughout their development the tooth germs move, relative to each other and relative to the developing bone of the jaw. Most of these motions appear to be somewhat random, the results of differential growth patterns inside the tooth germs.

Once most of the tooth crown has been formed and all crown odontoblasts and ameloblasts have differentiated, eruptive movements begin. *Eruptive movements* of a tooth consist of movements in a predominantly vertical direction, during which the crown of the tooth moves from its site of development inside the jaw to a position of functional occlusion in the oral cavity.

At some time during this eruption the tooth crown *emerges* through the oral epithelium into the oral cavity. This is what is commonly called tooth *eruption*. However, you should understand that eruption takes place over a long period of time and that the actual *emerging* of the tooth is only one episode in the stages of eruption.

The eruption from the developmental position inside the jaw to a position of functional occlusion inside the oral cavity is the result of real movements of the tooth relative to its environment and is called *prefunctional, active eruption*.

However, after the tooth has reached occlusion, wear of the occlusal or incisal surfaces may occur, and the tooth has to erupt a little bit more to maintain occlusal contact. This (minor) eruptive movement is called *functional, active eruption*.

Finally, with age, the gingiva recedes, usually exposing more of the tooth (clinical crown) than was originally exposed. Although the tooth seems to move up, relative to the gingiva, the actual movement is done by the gingiva, while the tooth remains in the same position. Such "eruption" of the tooth is called *passive eruption*.

While we are able to *describe* the appearances of the various stages of tooth eruption, until now no satisfactory explanation has been given for questions such as: "What makes a tooth erupt?" and "What constitutes the mechanism of the eruptive movements?"

Answers that have been considered are: the expansion of the dental papilla, the growth of the epithelial root sheath, bone deposition on the floor of the bony crypt, and the growth activities of the dental sac. At present, we believe that the answer to this question should be sought in some, as yet unknown, property of the dental sac.

At the start of the prefunctional, active eruption, the situation is as follows. The developing tooth is located in a bony crypt, which is a subdivision of the original, common, bony groove. All crown odontoblasts and all ameloblasts have differentiated, and several of these cells are still involved in the deposition of dentin and enamel.

In the incisal/occlusal part of the crown, dentin and enamel deposition are largely completed.

The outer enamel surface is covered with the collapsed remnants of the enamel organ, which together are called the reduced enamel epithelium. Cervically, the epithelial root sheath begins to proliferate, to start shaping the root.

As the tooth crown begins to move toward the oral epithelium, the inwardly curved edges of the bony crypt undergo bone resorption. This will allow the tooth crown to move freely out of the bony crypt. Once the bone opening is wide enough for the tooth to pass through, bone deposition takes place in a vertical direction (toward the oral mucosa) at the edges of the bony crypt. This is the beginning of the formation of the alveolar bone socket, in which the mature, functional tooth will be suspended.

Vertical movements of the crown toward the oral epithelium are possible, because the connective tissue between the oral epithelium and the reduced enamel epithelium is broken down and digested by the cells of the reduced enamel epithelium (Fig. 9–23).

Once the oral epithelium and the reduced enamel epithelium come together, fusion takes place between the 2 epithelia. The fused epithelia no longer have a blood supply, and as a result, the central cells perish, establishing an open path for the emergence of the tooth into the oral cavity.

When the tooth reaches its functional occlusion, the cervical part of the anatomical crown is still covered with reduced enamel epithelium. This epithelium is fused orally with the gingival epithelium. For some time after the tooth has started functioning, this remnant of the reduced enamel epithelium forms the first junction between the tooth and the gingiva. Only later will these epithelial cells be replaced by cells of the oral epithelium (Chap. 14).

Proliferation of the epithelial root sheath generally coincides with the eruptive movements of the tooth. Since the speed of the apical proliferation of the root sheath is approximately the same as the speed of the occlusal eruptive movements, the proliferating tip of the root sheath remains in about the same position, relative to the jaw bone.

When the speed of the eruptive movements exceeds that of the root sheath proliferation (usually temporarily), the entire developing tooth, including the tip of the root sheath, undergoes a net movement in occlusal direction. In such a case bone deposition on the floor of the bony crypt fills in the area vacated by the root tip.

When the speed of root sheath proliferation exceeds (temporarily) that of the eruptive movements, the root sheath proliferates deeper (further apically) into the bone of the jaw. Under those circumstances the bony crypt has to be enlarged, and this is accomplished by resorption of bone in the floor of the crypt.

fusion of OE & REE (handwritten)

Fig. 9–23. Histologic section through a molar tooth during active, prefunctional eruption. The reduced enamel epithelium (REE) has approached the oral epithelium (OE) closely, at the expense of the intervening tissues. (From Sicher, H., and DuBrul, E.L.: Oral Anatomy. 6th Ed. St. Louis, The C.V. Mosby Co., 1975.)

As we mentioned before, once the epithelial root sheath has shaped the root and has induced the differentiation of odontoblasts to form root dentin, the sheath falls apart into small cell rests of Malassez, without any further, apparent function. Some dental sac cells move between these cell rests and the root dentin, where they differentiate into cementoblasts.

The remaining dental sac cells differentiate into fibroblasts and begin to form the collagen fibers of the periodontal ligament. Other cells of the dental sac differentiate into osteoblasts and begin to form the inner walls of the alveolar socket of the tooth.

When the tooth reaches functional occlusion, about two-thirds of the length of its root(s) has (have) been formed. The root is still wide open apically; a thin layer of cementum has been deposited on its outer surface. Only the most cervical part of the periodontal ligament has been formed. The remainder of the root, its apical foramen, most of the cementum, the periodontal ligament and the alveolar bone are formed *after* the tooth has begun functioning.

Depending on the type of tooth, this may last another 1.5 to 3.5 years after functional occlusion has been reached (see timetables at the end of this chapter).

DEVELOPMENT AND ERUPTION OF THE SECONDARY DENTITION

Thus far we have discussed tooth development and eruption, limiting ourselves mainly to the developing primary dentition. Although the development and eruption of the teeth of the secondary dentition resemble these processes for the teeth of the primary dentition, a few differences should be noted.

The incisors, canines and premolars of the secondary dentition, which will replace elements of the primary dentition, first develop from tooth buds growing off the dental lamina, at the level of the tooth germs of the primary dentition, which are at that time in the bell stage. The secondary enamel organs remain temporarily attached to this parent dental lamina by a *successional dental lamina*. The secondary tooth germs form *lingual* to the primary tooth germs (Fig. 9–24).

The molars of the secondary dentition have *no* primary predecessors. Their enamel organs develop from a blind extension of the dental lamina of the primary dentition. This blind extension grows backward in the jaw, underneath the oral mucosa, from the dental lamina of the second molars of the primary dentition. This extension gives rise, in succession, to the enamel organs of the first, second and third molars of the secondary dentition (Fig. 9–25).

Once the tooth development of elements of the secondary dentition has been initiated, the development is essentially similar to that of the primary dentition.

Initially, the teeth of both dentitions develop at about the same vertical level: the primary teeth on the "outside," nearer the lips and cheeks, and the secondary teeth on the "inside," nearer the palate and the tongue. Also, all teeth are located within the same bony groove for a while, and later each primary tooth and its secondary successor share the same bony crypt (Fig. 9–26).

Once the primary teeth have erupted, the crowns of the secondary teeth are located on the lingual sides of the primary roots and, in some cases, even underneath these roots. Further bone development leads to the formation of separate bony sockets for the roots of

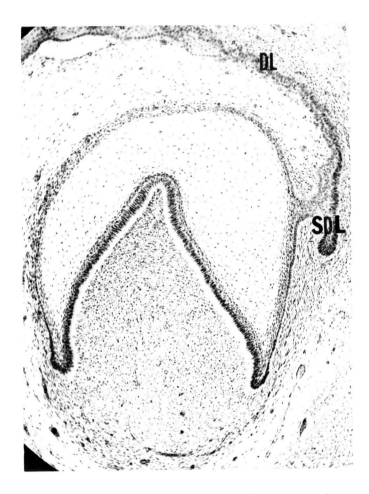

Fig. 9–24.   The early development of a successional dental lamina (SDL), as it appears in a histologic section, located lingual to the enamel organ (bell stage) of the primary tooth. DL = dental lamina. Original magnification × 20.

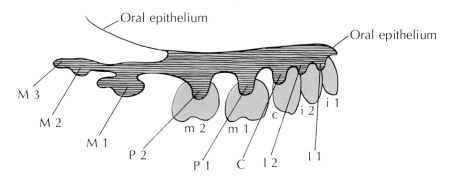

Fig. 9–25. A highly theoretical diagram (all components are not present at the same time) of the dental lamina and all enamel organs of primary and secondary dentitions in the left lower jaw, seen from the lingual side (inside). The primary enamel organs form after direct downgrowth of the dental lamina (darkly shaded) from the oral epithelium (indicated by a single line). The secondary successors of the primary teeth form from a successional dental lamina as localized further outgrowths of the dental lamina, lingual to the enamel organs of the primary teeth. The secondary molars develop from an extension of the dental lamina, growing backward underneath the oral epithelium.

Fig. 9–26. Relative positions, at various stages of development of a lower primary incisor and its secondary successor. A, Both teeth are located within a common bony crypt, at approximately the same vertical level. B, The primary tooth has become functional. Its root is located in a bony socket, while the secondary tooth is located in a separate bony crypt. During eruption of the secondary tooth, which is about to begin at this stage, the intervening connective tissues, the bone plate, which separates the crypt from the socket, and the root of the primary tooth must be resorbed. C, A newly erupted secondary incisor (the section has been reversed, so that the lingual side is now to the right). Bone remodeling has taken place to adapt the bony socket to this large new tooth. Original magnification A, × 2; B and C, × 1.

the primary teeth and bony crypts for the crowns of the secondary teeth.

While the secondary teeth are more completely enclosed by their bony crypts than the primary teeth ever were, a small occlusal opening is always present in the bony crypt wall containing the remnants of the successional dental lamina.

When the secondary teeth, except the molars, start their *eruption,* they not only have to remove some bone, connective tissue and epithelial cells, but also a more complete bony wall, a periodontal ligament and the root(s) of their predecessor. This is done, not only by the digestive abilities of the reduced enamel epithelium of the secondary teeth, but also by the differentiation of bone-resorbing cells *(osteoclasts)* and cementum and dentin-resorbing cells (multinucleated cells, resembling the osteoclasts in both appearance and function).

This process of resorption takes place slowly. First the wall of the bony crypt and part of the socket of the primary tooth are broken down. Cementum resorption at the surface of the root of the primary tooth follows, first and mostly on the side that faces the erupting secondary tooth.

The eruption of the secondary tooth is *not* continuous once it has started. There are long rest periods during which the secondary

Table 9–1.   Stages in the Development of the Primary Dentition

Tooth		Enamel organ in the bell stage, just prior to dentin deposition. *(Age in weeks after conception)*	Crown formation completed. *(Age in months after birth)*	Root formation completed. *(Age in years/ months after birth)*
i_1	upper	10	1.5	2/9
	lower	11	2.5	2/9
i_2	upper	12	2.5	2/9
	lower	12	3	2/6
c	upper	14	9	3/7
	lower	14	8–9	3/7
m_1	upper	13–14	6	3/1
	lower	13–14	5–6	2/10
m_2	upper	15–16	11	3/11
	lower	15–16	8–11	3/6

Table 9–2. Stages in the Development of the Secondary Dentition

Tooth		Enamel organ in the bell stage, just prior to dentin deposition. (Age in months after conception)	Crown formation completed. (Age in years after birth)	Root formation completed. (Age in years after birth)
I_1	upper	7.0	3.3– 4.1	8.6– 9.8
	lower	7.0	3.4– 5.4	7.7– 8.6
I_2	upper	7.0	4.4– 4.9	9.6–10.8
	lower	7.0	3.1– 5.9	8.5– 9.6
C	upper	7.0	4.5– 5.8	11.2–13.3
	lower	7.0	4.0– 4.7	10.8–13.0
P_1	upper	7.0	6.3– 7.0	11.2–13.6
	lower	7.0	5 – 6	11.0–13.4
P_2	upper	7.0	6.6– 7.2	11.6–14.0
	lower	7.0	6.1– 7.1	11.7–14.3
M_1	upper	5.5	2.1– 3.5	9.3–10.8
	lower	5.5	2.1– 3.6	7.8– 9.8
M_2	upper	6 months after birth	6.9– 7.4	12.9–16.2
	lower	6 months after birth	6.2– 7.4	11.0–15.7
M_3	upper	6 years after birth	12.8–13.2	19.5–19.6
	lower	6 years after birth	12.0–13.7	20.0–20.8

Table 9–3.   Clinical *Emergence* of Teeth in the Oral Cavity

---

Primary teeth:	i_1	upper :	9.1–10.6 months after birth
		lower :	7.3– 8.7 ″ ″ ″
	i_2	upper :	10.4–12.3 ″ ″ ″
		lower :	13.0–14.4 ″ ″ ″
	c	upper :	18.9–20.2 ″ ″ ″
		lower :	19.3–20.2 ″ ″ ″
	m_1	upper :	14.4–16.1 ″ ″ ″
		lower :	15.6–16.4 ″ ″ ″
	m_2	upper :	24.8–29.4 ″ ″ ″
		lower :	23.4–27.1 ″ ″ ″

Secondary teeth:	I_1	upper :	6.7– 8.1 years after birth
		lower :	6.0– 6.9 ″ ″ ″
	I_2	upper :	7.0– 8.8 ″ ″ ″
		lower :	6.8– 8.1 ″ ″ ″
	C	upper :	10.0–12.2 ″ ″ ″
		lower :	9.2–11.4 ″ ″ ″
	P_1	upper :	9.6–10.9 ″ ″ ″
		lower :	9.6–11.5 ″ ″ ″
	P_2	upper :	10.2–11.4 ″ ″ ″
		lower :	10.1–12.1 ″ ″ ″
	M_1	upper :	6.1– 6.7 ″ ″ ″
		lower :	5.9– 6.9 ″ ″ ″
	M_2	upper :	11.9–12.8 ″ ″ ″
		lower :	11.2–12.2 ″ ″ ″
	M_3	:	17 –19 ″ ″ ″

---

tooth may even move somewhat backward, allowing some repair-cementum to be formed in the resorption cavities of the primary root. Ultimately, however, the secondary tooth returns and more resorption of the primary root takes place.

These alternating periods of resorption, rest and repair, and new resorption continue until the entire root of the primary tooth has been resorbed. The crown of the primary tooth now falls out (the tooth is "shed") and the secondary tooth is able to erupt without further obstacles (Fig. 9–26).

TIMETABLES

Tables 9–1, 9–2 and 9–3 show the development and eruption of primary and secondary dentitions. Please remember that these dates are averages and that individuals may show a certain amount of variation without being abnormal. Nevertheless, these timetables, which should *not* be memorized, should give you some basic reference list to judge the state of development of a dentition in the dental practice (Figs. 9–27 and 9–28).

Fig. 9–27. A series of positive prints of x-rays of part of the lower jaw at various stages of development of the primary and secondary dentitions. What would be white in an x-ray is black in these prints. In the top row (late fetal and early neonatal period), the developing primary teeth are still located in the bony crypts within the jaw. In the middle row (2 to 4 years of age), the second molar of the primary dentition has just erupted. The bottom row, representing the age of 6 to 7 years, shows the first molar of the secondary dentition emerging. The second molar is still located in its bony crypt. The central incisor, not visible in these x-rays, is erupting as well. Once some secondary teeth have emerged, we speak of a mixed dentition. Both primary and secondary teeth are simultaneously present. This condition lasts until about the age of 12 to 13 years.

Fig. 9–28.   *Comparison of an x-ray of the premolar-molar region and a histologic section through the same region in the lower jaw of a child about 12 years of age. Notice especially the appearance of the developing roots in first and second premolars (P₁ and P₂) and in the second molar (M₂) of the secondary dentition. Note also the radiopaque (white) outline of the walls of the bony crypts around the developing second premolar and the second and third molars. Original magnification × 1.*

SELECTED READING LIST

Gaunt, W.A., and Miles, A.E.W.: Fundamental aspects of tooth morphogenesis. In *Structural and Chemical Organization of Teeth*. Volume I. Edited by A.E.W. Miles. New York, Academic Press, 1967.

Kraus, B.S., and Jordan, R.E.: *The Human Dentition Before Birth*. Philadelphia, Lea & Febiger, 1965.

Nery, E.B., Kraus, B.S., and Croup, M.: Timing and topography of early human tooth development. Arch. Oral Biol., *15*:1315, 1970.

Ooë, T.: On the development of position of the tooth germs in the human deciduous front teeth. Okaj. Folia Anat. Jap., *28*:317, 1956.

Ooë, T.: On the early development of human dental lamina. Okaj. Folia Anat. Jap. *30*:197, 1957.

Ooë, T.: On the development of position of the tooth germs in the human deciduous molar teeth. Okaj. Folia Anat. Jap., *32*:97, 1959.

Ooë, T.: On the development of position of the human deciduous molar germs in the latter half of fetal life. Okaj. Folia Anat. Jap., *38*:51, 1962.

Ooë, T.: On the position changes during development of human permanent tooth germs in the fetal life. Okaj. Folia Anat. Jap., *41*:1, 1965.

Ooë, T.: Changes in positions of deciduous molar and premolar germs during development. Okaj. Folia Anat. Jap., *44*:83, 1968.

Ooë, T.: Patterns of crowding of the anterior tooth germs in the fetal life. Okaj. Folia Anat. Jap., *45*:1, 1968.

Ooë, T.: Development of human first and second permanent molars with special reference to the distal portion of the dental lamina. Anat. Embryol., *155*:221, 1979.

Provenza, D. V., and Sisca, R. F.: Electron microscopic study of human dental primordia. Arch. Oral Biol., *16*:121, 1971.

Saxén, L., Karkinen-Jääskeläinen, M., Lehtonen, E., Nordling, S., and Wartiovaara, J.: Inductive tissue interactions. In *The Cell Surface in Animal Embryogenesis and Development*. Edited by G. Poste and G. L. Nicolsen. Amsterdam, Elsevier/North Holland Biomed. Press, 1976.

Slavkin, H.C.: Embryonic tooth formation. A tool for developmental biology. Oral Sciences Reviews, *4*:1, 1974.

Slavkin, H.C., and Bringas, P.: Epithelio-mesenchymal interactions during odontogenesis. IV. Morphological evidence for direct heterotypic cell-to-cell contacts. Developm. Biol., *50*:428, 1976.

Thesleff, I., Lehtonen, E., Wartiovaara, J., and Saxén, L.: Interference of tooth differentiation with interposed filters. Developm. Biol., *58*:197, 1977.

Van der Linden, F.P.G.M., and Duterloo, H.S.: *Development of the Human Dentition. An Atlas*. Hagerstown, Harper and Row, 1976.

The *timetables* of *dental development* were based on data from:

Fass, E.N.: J. Dent. Child., *36*:391, 1969.

Haavikko, K.: Suom. Hammaslääk. Toim., *66*:107, 1970.

Hurme, V.O.: J. Dent. Child., *16*:11, 1949.

Knott, V.B., and Meredith, H.V.: Angle Orthod., *36*:68, 1966.

Lunt, R.C., and Law, D.B.: JADA, *89*:872, 1974.

Lysell, L., Magnusson, B., and Thilander, B.: Odont. Revy, *13*:217, 1962.

Moorrees, C.F.A., Fanning, E.A., and Hunt, E.E.: Am. J. Phys. Anthrop., *21*:205, 1963.

Moorrees, C.F.A., Fanning, E.A., and Hunt, E.E.: J. Dent. Res., *42*:1490, 1963.

Nomata, N.: Bull. Tokyo Med. Dent. Univ., *11*:55, 1964.

Robinow, M., Richards, T.W., and Anderson, M.: Growth, *6*:127, 1942.

Röse, C.: Dtsch. Monatschr. Zahnheilk., *27*:553, 1909.

Schopf, P.M.: Fortschr. Kieferorthop., *31*:39, 1970.

Scott, J.H., and Symons, N.B.B.: Introduction to Dental Anatomy. 8th Ed. Edinburgh, Churchill/Livingstone, 1977.

Stones, H.H., Lawton, F.E., Bransby, E.R., and Hartley, H.O.: Brit. Dent. J., 90:1, 1951.

Tegzes, E.: Acta Paed. Hung., 1:289, 1960.

Turner, E.P.: Arch. Oral Biol., 8:523, 1963.

Chapter 10

PULP AND DENTIN

Developmentally and functionally, pulp and dentin are closely related, as they are both products of the *dental papilla* (which, in turn, is derived from neural crest cells).

During tooth development, the peripheral cells of the dental papilla differentiate to become odontoblasts. These cells produce dentin while moving backward, toward the center of the dental papilla. Whatever remains of the dental papilla after the dentin has been formed is transformed into the dental pulp.

Dentin and pulp form the core of any tooth. The *pulp* is the most centrally located tissue. It is enclosed entirely within the dentin, except at the *apical foramen*. The blood vessels and nerves of the pulp pass through this foramen, thus allowing some communication between the pulp and the tissues surrounding the tooth.

Clinically, this contact is important. A disease of the pulp tissue, most commonly inflammation, may spread through the apical foramen to the tissues of the periodontal ligament and to part of the alveolar bone. If the bone is affected, it will be resorbed. In x-ray films the effect of such resorption is visible as a dark area around the root tip, thus alerting you to the problem.

However, the patient usually has sought help before the problem gets this far. The pulp has the ability to cause excruciating pain. Because of this, people sometimes call the pulp the nerve(s) of the tooth, although in fact only a small part of the volume of the pulp consists of nerves. The pulp is a loose connective tissue, with particular characteristics, due to its unusual location, inside a shell of dentin (Fig. 10–1).

Any time dentin is exposed to the oral cavity, an open connection is established between the oral cavity and the pulp tissue, via a large number of open *dentinal tubules*. All stimuli reaching the pulp (heat, cold, pressure) are translated as *pain* by this tissue.

In young healthy teeth *dentin* is *not* ordinarily exposed to the oral cavity. There are, however, certain situations in which dentin may become exposed. On those occasions, when this does occur, the experience frequently is a quite painful one.

Fig. 10–1. Histologic section through the anatomical crown of a young, newly erupted premolar. The enamel cap has been lost during histologic processing. Only the organic contents of the occlusal fissure (arrow) remain. The darkly staining dentin (D) forms a shell of calcified tissue around the dental pulp (P) in the pulp chamber. The pulp is a highly vascularized, loose connective tissue (proper) organ. Original magnification × 5.

1. Dentin may be exposed as the result of *wear.* During occlusal function, enamel is gradually and slowly worn away at the cusps or incisal edges. Dentin, uncovered this way, is generally *not* painful, because the wearing process is slow. This enables the tooth to produce *reactive dentin* (see section on aging phenomena in this chapter). Reactive dentin seals off the pulpal openings of the exposed dentinal tubules, thus reducing the possibility of pain.

2. Dentin may be exposed as the result of *caries* or *trauma.* If the caries process is sufficiently slow, reactive dentin may be produced, minimizing the pain until the caries reaches the pulp and the pain becomes serious. When caries spreads rapidly or, in the case of trauma, when part of the tooth is broken off, the acutely exposed dentin may be exquisitely painful.

3. Some dentin may remain exposed because it is never covered with either enamel or cementum during *development*. Aside from some specific diseases, this situation occurs at the cervix of about 10% of all teeth (see a more extensive description in Chap. 14). In a young individual, such an area is covered with the tissues of the dentogingival junction, but as these tissues recede with age, the uncovered dentin is exposed to the oral cavity, causing frequently "painful necks of teeth" in older patients.

DENTAL PULP

The dental pulp is a *loose connective tissue* with components commonly found in connective tissues (Fig. 10–2):

1. *Cells*—fibroblasts and undifferentiated mesenchymal cells; other cell types required for the maintenance and defense of the tissue, specifically histiocytes and lymphocytes.

2. *Fibrous matrix*—reticulin fibers and some collagen fibers.

3. *Ground substance*—long carbohydrate chains, attached to protein "backbones." The ground substance contains large amounts of water and is chemically similar to the ground substance

Fig. 10–2. Peripheral pulp tissue in the anatomical crown of a young, newly erupted premolar. At the periphery of the pulp, a layer of odontoblasts (O) is located, each with a cytoplasmic process extending into a dentinal tubule. The dentinal tubules appear as dark lines in the dentin. The darkly staining structures inside the pulp tissue are blood vessels filled with red blood cells. The finest branches of these vessels are near the odontoblast layer. A nerve (N) is visible in the very delicate fibrous matrix of the pulp. The presence of a large number of cells is characteristic for young pulp tissue (see section on aging, this chapter). Original magnification × 40.

in other loose connective tissues, with only minor variations in the relative proportions of the ground substance components.

Compared with other connective tissues proper, the dental pulp should be regarded as a somewhat immature connective tissue. This is based on the relatively large proportion of *reticulin fibers* and the small proportion of *collagen fibers*. (Also, there seem to be relatively more undifferentiated mesenchymal cells.) No elastic fibers or oxytalan fibers are present in the dental pulp.

The cell population in the dental pulp consists, to a large extent, of *fibroblasts* and *undifferentiated mesenchymal cells*. The relatively large numbers of the latter enable the pulp to recruit newly differentiating cells to replace others when they are lost, specifically the odontoblasts. As we stated before, odontoblasts, once differentiated, no longer are capable of mitoses, and if groups of odontoblasts are lost, undifferentiated cells must be mobilized to replace them.

Along the blood vessels, *histiocytes* are found. These cells are capable of digestive activities. When they are well filled with ingested material, they are called *macrophages*.

In connective tissue proper, mast cells are generally present. As we stated earlier (Chap. 4), mast cells contain vesicles filled with heparin and histamine. When heparin is released by the cell, it prevents blood clotting, while the release of histamine causes a widening of the blood vessels. *Mast cells* are usually present in *inflamed* human pulps, but surprisingly have *not* been found in healthy human pulp tissue.

Of the wandering cells, which may be present in connective tissue proper, the only group of cells frequently seen in dental pulps are the *lymphocytes*. When present, they tend to be localized near the odontoblast layer, at the periphery.

The presence in the pulp of monocytes, polymorphonuclear leukocytes, eosinophils and plasma cells generally is indicative of disease. *No fat cells* are found in the dental pulp.

Vascularization and Innervation

Both the vascularization and innervation patterns of the dental pulp underscore the primary function of this tissue: the *support* and *maintenance* of the *odontoblast layer* at its periphery. The odontoblasts, in turn, maintain the dentin (Fig. 10–3).

Blood vessels (and nerves) enter the pulp via the apical foramen. One or more small arterioles enter and run in a fairly straight course through the pulp in the root canal. Once they reach the pulp chamber in the crown, they branch out, forming a rich capillary network at the periphery immediately underneath, and occasionally within, the layer of odontoblasts. The odontoblast layer is active metabolically, and the capillaries near the odontoblasts have many

Fig. 10–3.   Diagrammatic representation of the vascular pattern of a dental pulp. A similar pattern exists for the nerves of the pulp. Arteries enter the pulp and veins leave the pulp via the apical foramen (as do the nerves). They run through the root canal, where they give off relatively few branches. In the pulp chamber of the crown a profuse branching takes place. The microvasculature of the pulp is associated with the odontoblast layer. Similarly, the richly branching afferent nerves form a fine network (plexus) near the odontoblast layer.

pores (see Chap. 6); consequently there is extensive exchange of materials across the capillary wall.

Drainage from the capillary bed is by several small venules, which come together into 2 or 3 larger venules, running back toward the apical foramen.

It is difficult to demonstrate satisfactorily the presence of lymph capillaries in the dental pulp. A few investigators have provided some morphologic evidence for such vessels. However, others claim that no lymph capillaries are found in the dental pulp. If the latter claim is correct, fluid from the ground substance, which in most other tissues returns to the blood via the lymph capillaries, must take a different pathway in the pulp, perhaps directly back into the blood capillaries. Unless such an alternative mechanism is in fact demonstrated, it seems reasonable to assume that lymph capillaries do exist in the dental pulp.

Two types of *nerve fibers* enter the dental pulp via the apical foramen: autonomic and afferent.

AUTONOMIC NERVE FIBERS. Only sympathetic autonomics are found in the pulp. The fibers consist of the cell processes of those neurons whose cell bodies are located in the superior cervical ganglion. These *unmyelinated* nerve fibers travel along with the blood vessels. Their function in the pulp is the innervation of the smooth muscle cells of the arterioles and thus the regulation of the *blood flow* in the *microvascular bed.*

AFFERENT (SENSORY) FIBERS. These fibers come from branches of the second and third divisions of the fifth cranial (trigeminal) nerve. These *mostly myelinated* fibers initially run along with the blood vessels into the pulp chamber of the crown. There they branch out and break up into small individual fibers. The fibers form a rich network (*plexus* of *Raschkow*) underneath the odontoblastic layer. From this plexus, individual nerve fibers run peripherally toward the odontoblastic layer. These nerve fibers are no longer covered with a myelin sheath; they consist of axons, supported by Schwann cells.

The nerve fibers finally lose their Schwann cell cover and terminate as *"free endings."* This is the only type of afferent nerve terminal in the dental pulp. The free ending may touch the cell body of an odontoblast, or it may run for a short distance inside the dentinal tubule and terminate on the odontoblastic process. Most odontoblasts are *not* associated with such free nerve endings, but since the odontoblasts are connected with each other via gap junctions and/or tight junctions, a sheet of these cells behaves as an organic unit, so that individual innervation is not required. The presence of free nerve endings is held responsible for the perception of *pain* by the dental pulp of all stimuli, regardless of the nature of these stimuli (heat, cold, pressure, Fig. 10–4).

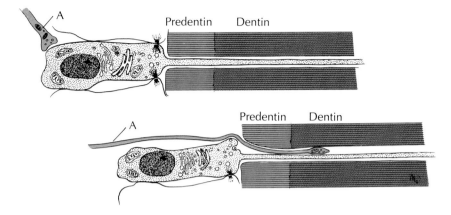

Fig. 10–4. This diagram shows afferent nerve endings on 2 odontoblasts. The axon (A) has lost its Schwann cell support, just before reaching the odontoblast layer. The axon may terminate in close association with the odontoblast's cell body (top), or it may run for a short distance inside a dentinal tubule and terminate on an odontoblastic process (bottom). The nerve terminals somewhat resemble a synapse.

DENTIN

Dentin, somewhat comparable to bone tissue, has the 3 components commonly found in connective tissues: *cells* (odontoblasts), *fibrous matrix* (collagen fibers) and *ground substance* (long carbohydrate chains, attached to protein "backbones" chemically somewhat similar to the ground substance of bone).

The dominant component of this tissue is the fibrous matrix. Dentin is calcified, which means that hydroxyapatite salts are present in the fibrous matrix and ground substance.

Dentin is morphologically unique in that the odontoblasts do *not* become *enclosed* by their product, except for one long cell process, which each of these cells leaves behind in the dentin.

The cell bodies of the odontoblasts are located in the dental pulp at the inner surface of the dentin. Their long cell processes are surrounded by dentin matrix (calcified in the mature dentin, uncalcified in the immature predentin), so that each process lies in its individual *dentinal tubule*. All dentinal tubules run from the dentino-enamel junction to the dental pulp.

Once dentin is exposed by a carious lesion, trauma or otherwise, there is a direct contact between the outside world and the dental pulp, via a large number of patent dentinal tubules. This contact is usually experienced as extremely unpleasant and painful.

Dentinal Tubules

It would be possible to fill several pages with the many histologic details of dentin, but from a clinical viewpoint the most important attributes of this tissue are its dentinal tubules.

COURSE OF THE DENTINAL TUBULES: S-SHAPED CURVATURES. As we stated before, the dentinal tubules are formed as the result of deposition of dentin *around* the odontoblastic cell processes which, during dentin formation, are left behind by the odontoblasts. Since the odontoblastic processes are left behind while the odontoblasts are moving backward, the shape of the odontoblastic processes and of the dentinal tubules in which they are located provide us with an accurate record of the path taken by the odontoblasts.

In analyzing a longitudinal section of a tooth, you will soon recognize that in a large part of the tooth the dentinal tubules are not straight, but rather gently curved in an ·S-shape.

The peculiar course of the dentinal tubules is explained when you realize that, during the deposition of the dentin matrix, the odonto-blasts move backward toward the center of the dental papilla. This means that the cells start out on a larger surface and end up occupying a much smaller surface. If both the original surface and the later surface would be perfectly spherical, the cells would all move centrally in a straight line while becoming increasingly more densely packed.

However, the particular shape of a tooth, that of a fairly straight cylinder, with cusps or an incisal edge on one end, forces the odontoblasts to move in a slightly more complicated manner. In the roots, which are mostly cylindrically shaped, the dentinal tubules run relatively straight. In the crown, on the other hand, uneven and locally acute crowding patterns would develop if the odontoblasts would all try to move straight backward during their secretory activity.

They do so, but only for a short distance. Thereafter they move obliquely in an apical direction, producing an S-shaped curve and thus making accommodations for the more occlusally/incisally located odontoblasts. In this way, while the odontoblasts do become densely packed, the crowding is at least evenly divided (Fig. 10–5).

For survival, the odontoblastic cell bodies, which were arranged in a single layer at the start of their secretory activities, rearrange themselves into several layers, up to 8 layers in the crown.

The S-shaped curvature of the dentinal tubules in the crown and cervical region of the tooth has clinical significance. Caries, or any other external insult that affects the peripheral dentin, may have a local effect in the dental pulp at a more apical level than the level at which the external insult occurred. Conversely, if a stained, pig-

Fig. 10-5. Early crowding patterns in the odontoblast layer (O) during dentin formation. The orientation of the odontoblastic cell bodies forms an angle with the orientation of the first-formed parts of the dentinal tubules in the dentin (D). Since the odontoblasts will move further backward in a direction, corresponding with the orientation of their cell bodies, the first part of an (inverted) S-curve is about to be formed. Original magnification × 125.

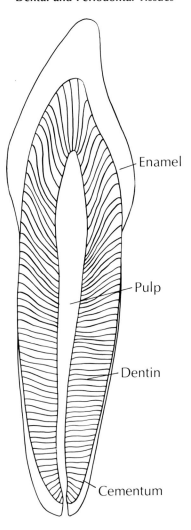

Fig. 10–6.　Simplified diagram showing the course of the dentinal tubules, indicated with lines, inside the dentin. In the crown dentin and the dentin near the cervix, the dentinal tubules run in an S-shaped course, while further apically, in the root dentin, the tubules straighten out and become horizontal.

mented endodontic filling has been placed above a certain level in the root canal, but still below the level of the cervix, discoloration of the dentin in the crown may follow nonetheless, since the pigments travel in occlusal/incisal direction, upward along the S-shaped dentinal tubules (Fig. 10–6).

　　SECONDARY CURVATURES OF THE DENTINAL TUBULES. Careful microscopic study of the dentinal tubules may reveal the presence of a finer pattern of delicate curves, or *secondary curvatures,* along their course. These curvatures consist of small waves in the dentinal tubules, with crests about 4 μm apart.

They probably reflect the minor changes in the direction of movement of the dentin-producing odontoblasts during the day and night.

DENSITY AND BRANCHING OF THE DENTINAL TUBULES. An odontoblastic process and the tubule in which it lies reflect the path taken by the odontoblast during dentin deposition. Since the odontoblasts become progressively more crowded as they move toward the center of the dental papilla, it is easy to understand that the dentinal tubules are closer together in the dentin near the pulp than in the peripheral dentin. In fact, if one were to count the total number of cross-sectioned tubules in 1 mm² of dentin (in a section), as a measure of tubular *density,* this density would be 4 to 5 times higher in the dentin near the pulp than in the peripheral dentin.

At the dentino-enamel junction, however, the tubule density becomes suddenly higher than in the rest of the peripheral dentin. This is because the terminal parts of the dentinal tubules, near the dentino-enamel junction, are branched into 2 or 3 short branches. This higher tubular density makes this part of the dentin sensitive on exposure, almost as sensitive as the dentin near the pulp.

The terminal branching of the dentinal tubules is produced during the earliest stages of dentin formation. At that time the odontoblasts have several cell processes, some of which contact the processes of the pre-ameloblasts across the broken-down basal lamina (see Chap. 9). As the odontoblasts recede, the original processes come together into one single odontoblastic process. The dentin is first deposited around the larger number of smaller processes and later around the single process, producing the terminally branched dentinal tubule.

Aside from the terminal branching, the dentinal tubules in the crown dentin are relatively unbranched (Fig. 10–7). In the root dentin, however, the tubules have many side branches, all along their lengths. These side branches are also produced during dentin formation, and they are the result of cell junctions between the adjacent odontoblasts or additional small cell processes, which become trapped in the forming dentin.

DIAMETERS AND CONTENTS OF THE DENTINAL TUBULES. When dentinal tubules are first formed, during the process of dentin formation, they are wide, up to 4 μm in diameter. With further development, however, a small amount of dentin is added to the inner surfaces of the tubular walls. This reduces the diameters of these tubules somewhat.

The tubule diameter near the dentino-enamel junction is a little less than 2 μm and this does not change much with age. Midway

Fig. 10–7. Dentinal tubules in a ground section of crown dentin. In contrast with the tubules in root dentin, these tubules are relatively unbranched. Secondary curvatures are visible in some (asterisk). The presence of air, enclosed in one of the tubules during histologic processing, makes this tubule stand out (arrow). Original magnification × 600.

along the length of the dentinal tubules their diameter is 2.5 to 3 μm (the wider diameter is found in younger teeth). Near the pulp the dentinal tubules are widest: 3 to 4 μm (again, the wider diameters are in the younger teeth).

Inside a dentinal tubule, at least during the period of dentin formation, a long odontoblastic process is found. Soon after the dentin is formed, this process recedes a little, so that in a mature tooth the odontoblastic process fills only about one half (the half nearest the dental pulp) of the length of the dentinal tubule. The rest of the tubule is filled with tissue fluid, and occasionally with fat droplets or uncalcified collagen fibers.

In some dentinal tubules a delicate, afferent (sensory) nerve axon is present. This axon is not covered by a Schwann cell and it terminates on the odontoblastic process, which is located in the same tubule. If present, a nerve axon does *not* extend farther into the dentinal tubule than the odontoblastic process itself. The presence of an axon inside a dentinal tubule is probably explained by the fact that it became enclosed in the forming dentin, together with the odontoblastic process.

With age, the contents of those segments of the dentinal tubules that no longer contain part of the odontoblastic process may calcify. This is the case especially near the dentino-enamel junction.

At the beginning of this chapter, we described the possibility of having exposed dentin at the cervix of the tooth. When the dentin has been acutely exposed, the tubules form an open connection between the outside world and the dental pulp, thus causing a painful situation. However, if the contents of the dentinal tubules are calcified, they seal off the remainder of the tubular contents from the outside world. This, in turn, affords protection for the dental pulp, and little pain may be produced when such dentin is exposed. Certain clinical treatments for painful cervical dentin actually stimulate the calcification of the dentinal tubules, thereby reducing the pain.

Peritubular and Intertubular Dentin

Dentin (fibrous matrix, ground substance and the mineral hydroxyapatite) is not completely homogeneous. The dentin immediately around each dentinal tubule *(peritubular dentin)* differs in composition from the remainder of the dentin *(intertubular dentin)*.

Peritubular dentin forms a 1 μm thick sheath around each tubule. This sheath consists of a fibrous matrix of delicate collagen fibers, which, together with the ground substance, is heavily calcified.

In the *intertubular dentin* the collagen fibers are much coarser, and they occupy a certain volume that cannot be occupied by hydroxyapatite. Thus intertubular dentin has a far less delicate fibrous matrix and is less heavily calcified than peritubular dentin.

During dentin formation, the intertubular dentin is produced first. The protein-producing organelles (granular endoplasmic reticulum, Golgi systems) are all located in the odontoblastic cell body. The secretory granules, which contain the protein precursors of the collagen fibers and the proteins of the ground substance, to which carbohydrates have been added in the Golgi system, are secreted at the secretory end of the odontoblastic *cell body*. Thus, the odontoblastic processes *first* become surrounded by *intertubular dentin matrix*.

While this matrix undergoes calcification, some secretory granules move into the odontoblastic processes. The processes themselves do *not* contain any protein-synthesizing organelles, and their cytoplasm is relatively empty, apart from some microtubules and microfilaments, which give support to these long cell processes.

slightly less calcified

odontoblast

highly mineralized

Fig. 10–8. Diagram of an odontoblast with its cytoplasmic process extended into a dentinal tubule. A second, empty tubule appears below the first. Continued dentin deposition by the odontoblasts (secretory vesicles in the cell body) leads to the formation of more predentin, which calcifies and becomes (intertubular) dentin. During the calcification of the intertubular dentin matrix, additional dentin matrix is deposited (secretory vesicles in odontoblastic process) on the inside walls of the dentinal tubules. This is peritubular (darkly shaded) dentin, which has a different composition than the intertubular dentin and calcifies almost immediately. The layer of peritubular dentin reduces the diameter of the dentinal tubule substantially.

The secretory granules in the odontoblastic processes release their contents on the inside surfaces of the dentinal tubular walls, which still consist of intertubular dentin. The newly released materials form the matrix of the peritubular dentin, which calcifies almost as soon as it is deposited (Fig. 10–8).

The difference in composition between peritubular and intertubular dentin causes these 2 dentins to behave differently, notably during *decalcification*. When peritubular dentin is decalcified, its delicate fibrous matrix is disrupted completely and is lost. In decalcified histologic sections of dentin, only the decalcified matrix of intertubular dentin remains, and as a result, the tubules appear much wider than they are in the nondecalcified tooth. Compare the widths of the dentinal tubules in decalcified histologic sections and in ground sections of dentin and verify this statement (Fig. 10–9).

Clinically, whenever dentin is in contact with a decalcifying agent (even small amounts of acid, such as the acids produced by bacteria in carious dentin, or acids leaked out of the cement of a temporary filling), some peritubular dentin is lost, and the tubules become wider, giving even more access to the dental pulp and causing more pain.

Pain

Pain has been mentioned several times on the preceding pages. It is well known that exposed, healthy dentin, with open dentinal tubules, may be painful. The pain is severe at the dentino-enamel

Fig. 10–9.   Cross sectioned dentinal tubules in a ground section, A, and a decalcified histologic section, B. In the ground section the dentinal tubules have a narrow, dark lumen, surrounded by a bright "halo" of well-calcified peritubular dentin. Between the halos intertubular dentin is present. In the decalcified section the dentinal tubules appear to have a wider lumen. This is the result of the total loss of the peritubular dentin layer during decalcification. Only intertubular dentin remains. Original magnification × 125.

junction, less so in the middle of the dentin, and becomes more severe in the dentin nearest the pulp. The question, why dentin should be so painful, has been asked for a long time. Several answers have been given and some have been proven wrong.

Nerve endings do *not* run along the *entire* lengths of the dentinal tubules, nor do the odontoblastic processes. Therefore, the pain at the dentino-enamel junction *cannot* be explained by damage to these cell processes or by direct stimulation of the nerve endings.

The most likely explanation given to date is that the fluid present in the dentinal tubules evaporates when the tubules are opened. The movement of fluid in the tubules, which results from this evaporation, would stimulate the nerve axons, which terminate on some of the odontoblasts. These stimuli would be perceived as pain.

This explanation seems to fit most, if not all, clinical experiences, and while it is not completely accepted, it is at present the best available explanation for dentin pain.

Other Aspects of Dentin

For a good understanding of dentin in clinical practice, an understanding of the dentinal tubules, as well as of peritubular and intertubular dentin, is most important. However, the following points are of interest and we will discuss them briefly here.

Dentin, Once Deposited, Does Not Undergo Any Remodeling

Throughout life, some dentin deposition continues to take place, but except for the resorption of roots of primary teeth, which leads to the shedding of those teeth, resorption of dentin is an indication of a pathologic condition. This means that dentin provides us with a record of the events that occurred in the body during dentin deposition, somewhat like growth rings in a tree:

1. *IMBRICATION LINES* (von Ebner). The dentin deposited at night differs from that deposited during the daytime—in amount, nature of the matrix and degree of calcification of this matrix. Thus, if the daily deposition rate of dentin is about 4 μm, each 4 μm of dentin in a *ground section* is composed of a somewhat lighter (more calcified) and a somewhat darker (less calcified) band. In decalcified and stained histologic sections such bands, or lines, are visible as well (Fig. 10–10). These lines, representing alternate bands of dentin deposited during daytime and during nighttime, are called *imbrication lines* (von Ebner).

2. *CONTOUR LINES* (Owen). During periods of illness or other major changes in body metabolism (birth, for example), the dentin deposition may be somewhat affected as well. As a result, a band of dentin of a slightly different composition may be produced. Such a band is usually less well calcified than the adjacent dentin

~~contour~~ liney of ~~orden~~ Von Ebner

Fig. 10–10. Imbrication lines in a decalcified histologic section of a young, newly erupted premolar. Odontoblasts (O) line the pulpal surface of the dentin. Their cytoplasmic processes are located within the dentinal tubules, of which the lower part of the S-shaped curve is visible. The imbrication lines appear as very regular, alternately dark and light bands (arrows). Original magnification × 40.

(formed before and after) and shows as a darker band in ground sections of dentin. These bands, which are far less frequently present than imbrication lines, are called *contour lines* (Owen). They follow the contour of what used to be the pulpal surface of the forming dentin at the time of the disturbance or change (Fig. 10–11). Since only the teeth of the primary dentition and the first molars of the secondary dentition are involved in dentin production at the time of birth, a clear *neonatal line* (a pronounced contour line) is present only in the dentin of these teeth.

   MAN-MADE CONTOUR LINES. Certain antibiotics, most notably tetracyclines, are chemically bound to matrix components and even more to hydroxyapatite at the *growing surfaces* of bone, cementum and dentin.

   Bone and cementum are well embedded in soft tissues, so that any discoloration of these 2 tissues, as the result of the binding of tetracycline, remains undetected. Furthermore, bone is constantly remodeled and so, in time, rids itself of the tetracycline. But dentin is permanently marked because the tetracycline remains fixed in this nonremodeling tissue for the life of the tooth. Since the tetracycline attaches itself to the components of the forming dentin, along what is the pulpal surface of the dentin at the time of the

Lines of Owen

Fig. 10–11. Ground section through the anatomical crown of an incisor. Several dark contour lines (Owen) are visible in the dentin (arrows). Each of these lines represents the position of the odontoblast layer at the time of the insult, which produced that particular line. Original magnification × 2.5.

tetracycline administration, the band of stained dentin has the same shape as a contour line. Tetracycline has a deep golden color. Enamel is a transparent tissue. This is especially evident in areas where the enamel layer is thin, as it is near the cervix of the tooth. If stained dentin is located in the crown, a dark band may be visible through the enamel. As a result, the tooth becomes esthetically unattractive. Although it is possible to bleach such teeth somewhat, the tetracycline remains. It cannot be removed.

Not All Dentin Calcifies Perfectly

Occasionally, during dentin matrix calcification, small islands of dentin matrix remain uncalcified. In number and size, these non-calcified regions vary from individual to individual. They are imperfections in calcification, but generally are *not* considered pathologic, since most teeth have them.

Once the imperfections are present, they usually do *not* disappear. With age, some minerals may diffuse into such areas and become deposited in them. This makes these areas somewhat better, but by no means perfectly, calcified. We distinguish 2 types of imperfections in dentin calcification:

Fig. 10–12. Horizontal ground sections through the crown, A, and the root, B, of a human tooth. In the crown dentin interglobular dentin areas are present (dark structures). The granular layer (Tomes) is found in the root dentin, in the most peripheral layer, immediately adjacent to the (acellular) cementum, C. In both sections, the less calcified dentin areas have been stained with a dye, to make them more clearly visible. A, The rounded surfaces of well-calcified dentin globules demarcate the less calcified interglobular dentin areas. The granules of the granular layer (Tomes) have similar shapes, but are considerably smaller. Original magnification × 50.

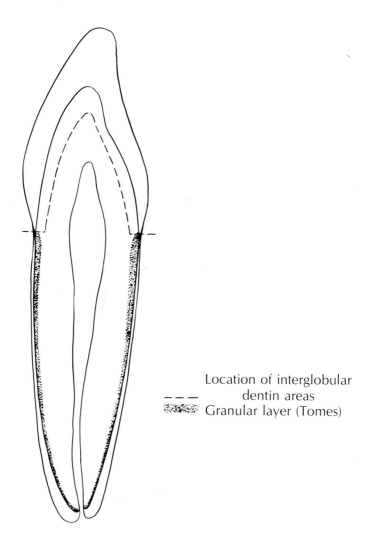

Location of interglobular
dentin areas
Granular layer (Tomes)

Fig. 10–13.   Diagram illustrating the principal locations of interglobular dentin areas and the granular layer (Tomes) in a section of a human tooth. The interglobular dentin areas generally are located in the crown dentin, along a line between outer third and middle third of the dentin width (where the dentinal tubules make their first curve of the S-shape). The granular layer is found in the most peripheral dentin of the root only.

INTERGLOBULAR DENTIN AREAS. These small islands of dentin, which are somewhat or not at all calcified, are located in the crown. They are found mostly along the line between the outer third and the middle third of the dentin width. Since the dentin calcifies in spheres, the calcified dentin around these areas consists of spheres or globules, and thus the *interglobular areas* have rounded depressions in their outer surface.

GRANULAR LAYER (Tomes). In the most peripheral dentin of the root, multitudes of noncalcified dentin islands are present, appearing as dark grains immediately next to the dentinocementum junction, in ground sections. These islands have the same shapes as the interglobular dentin areas, but they are considerably smaller (Figs. 10–12 and 10–13).

Mantle Dentin and Circumpulpal Dentin

Although most dentin is called _circumpulpal_ (around the pulp), the _outermost layer_ of the _crown_ dentin, immediately next to the dentino-enamel junction, is called _mantle dentin._ This layer is about 10 to 30 μm thick. It is different from the circumpulpal dentin, because it contains, *in addition* to the normal collagen fibers of the dentin, another group of collagen fibers, which are considerably thicker. These thicker fibers are called *von Korff's* fibers. The normal collagen fibers run parallel to the dentino-enamel junction. The von Korff's fibers run nearly perpendicular to the dentino-enamel junction.

In the section on peritubular and intertubular dentin, we noted that a fibrous matrix of thick collagen fibers is *less* calcified than a matrix with more delicate fibers. The same is true for mantle dentin. It is somewhat less calcified than the circumpulpal dentin because of the presence of the heavy von Korff's fibers. This lesser degree of calcification may explain the spread of caries along the dentino-enamel junction, once this junction is reached by the caries process.

AGE CHANGES AND PATHOLOGIC CHANGES IN DENTIN AND PULP

Pulp

In the pulp certain changes occur with age. Cell death results in a *decrease* in the number of cells. The surviving fibroblasts gradually produce *more fibrous matrix,* with an increased proportion of collagen fibers, at the expense of the reticulin fibers. *Less ground substance* is produced, and the ground substance contains *less water.* Thus, with age, the pulp becomes less cellular and more fibrous. In addition, the actual *size* of the pulp *decreases* as a result of further dentin deposition (p. 225).

Occasionally small calcified bodies are present in a dental pulp. These are called *denticles*. We distinguish 3 types: *true* denticles, *false* denticles and *diffuse calcifications*.

TRUE DENTICLES. True denticles are generally formed during tooth formation and are usually found in the root canals of a tooth. It is not clear what causes the production of such denticles. They probably develop when a small clump of epithelial cells breaks loose from the epithelial root sheath, during root development. In any case, whatever the cause, centrally located dental papilla cells are induced and differentiate into odontoblasts. These odontoblasts then produce a small body of dentin inside the pulp, complete with dentinal tubules and lined at the periphery with odontoblastic cell bodies.

True denticles are defined morphologically by the presence of dentinal tubules and the odontoblasts at their periphery. This distinguishes them from false denticles (Fig. 10–14).

FALSE DENTICLES. False denticles usually are formed at a later age and frequently in the crown pulp. They start forming when a component of the pulp tissue—a collagen fiber, some ground substance, a dead cell, part of a capillary—undergoes spontaneous calcification. This small calcified structure may continue to grow in an *irregular* fashion by calcification of the structures surrounding the original site of calcification (Fig. 10–15).

Fig. 10–14. Large true denticle in a histologic section through the root pulp of a human tooth. Some irregular dentinal tubules (arrow) are visible inside the denticle, and odontoblasts (O) line those parts of the denticle, which contain the dentinal tubules. Original magnification × 50.

pulp stones or false denticles (handwritten annotation)

Fig. 10–15.   Several false denticles are present in this histologic section (decalcified) of a molar tooth of an older individual. Notice the extensive caries at the cervix and an old cavity on the right side. Some of the denticles have a regular, lamellar appearance (arrows). Others have an irregular appearance (and are darker in this section). Original magnification × 1.

The initially calcified mass may induce certain cells in the pulp to become osteoblast-like cells. These differentiated cells then produce layer upon concentric layer of a calcifying matrix. In contrast with the irregularly calcifying, false denticle, this calcification is regular. No cells are enclosed in this matrix.

DIFFUSE CALCIFICATIONS. A seriously ill pulp may undergo spontaneous calcifications in a large number of locations. This is called diffuse calcification. Morphologically a diffuse calcification resembles irregular false denticles. The difference between the 2 is that there are large numbers of calcified masses in a diffuse calcification, while a false denticle may be all by itself (Fig. 10–16).

Pulp calcifications may be visible on dental x-ray films. Some may cause problems, especially the false denticles and the diffuse calcifications. The true denticles may not give any problems because of their slow growth.

Fig. 10–16. *Evidence of diffuse calcification in this histologic section of the root pulp of a human tooth. Dark, tiny areas of diffuse calcification are visible. Most appear to be related to existing structures, such as collagen fibers and blood vessels. Original magnification × 12.5.*

Because of their continued growth and because of the dentin production by the regular odontoblasts along the pulpal walls, the denticles, which generally begin as *loose* denticles inside the pulp tissue, may become *attached* denticles (attached to the dentin walls), or they may even become *embedded* denticles (embedded within the dentin walls). Usually, only true denticles become embedded.

Dental pulp tissue is somewhat unique, mainly because it is surrounded by hard tissues. Because of its location, *minor pathologic events,* such as an inflammation, may have far-reaching effects. Inflammation is usually accompanied by a swelling of the affected tissue. Elsewhere in the body this does not lead to complications. However, a dental pulp is not capable of undergoing swelling because the surrounding hard tissues prevent its expansion. Since there is no place to accommodate an increase in dimension of this tissue, it becomes compressed. This can cause extreme pain, and in severe cases, it leads to the loss of the inflamed pulp.

Dentin

As we stated before, dentin production continues throughout the functional life of the tooth. All dentin formed *before* the completion of the apical foramen is considered *primary dentin*. Once the apical foramen is completed, dentin formation continues, but at a considerably slower rate. This dentin is *secondary dentin*.

Morphologically, secondary dentin may be recognized by an abrupt *change* in the *course* of the dentinal tubules, at the transition between primary and secondary dentin. Also, there is a slight *reduction* in the *number* of the dentinal tubules that can be explained only by the cell death of some of the odontoblasts, at the completion of the primary dentin. Finally, the secondary dentin *matrix* is somewhat *more calcified* than the primary dentin matrix (Fig. 10–17).

Secondary dentin is not formed evenly along all dentin walls of the pulp. It is formed mostly on those dentin surfaces that are underneath functionally loaded surfaces of the tooth, such as the lingual surfaces of incisors and canines.

REACTIVE DENTIN. This type of dentin is also frequently, and inappropriately, called reparative dentin. However, it does not really repair anything. Reactive dentin is formed fast and in localized regions, involving only the areas underneath those dentinal tubules that are exposed to some external insult. The insult may be caries, a cavity preparation, or dentin exposed following excessive wear of the enamel.

In all these cases a localized group of odontoblasts related to the tubules that are affected by the insult may perish. If odontoblasts

Fig. 10–17.　Primary (P), secondary (S) and reactive (R) dentin in a ground section of a human tooth. The difference between primary and secondary dentin is primarily due to the slight change in the course of the dentinal tubules, as they pass from the primary into the secondary dentin, and to a somewhat higher degree of calcification of the secondary dentin (lighter in ground section). The reactive dentin is associated with wear of the cusps, which has exposed part of the dentin (not visible in this photograph). The dentinal tubules in the reactive dentin are irregular and smaller in number than in primary and secondary dentin. Original magnification × 10.

perish, neighboring undifferentiated, mesenchymal cells move to the affected dentin and become odontoblasts. These cells produce a small, localized patch of reactive dentin.

The new tissue has irregular dentinal tubules and occasionally no tubules at all. Sometimes odontoblasts become trapped in this dentin.

The dentinal tubules, which run between the dentino-enamel junction and this new patch of reactive dentin, usually no longer contain any odontoblastic processes. These processes are lost when the odontoblasts themselves perish. During the preparation of a ground section, such empty tubules may fill up with air. Because of the presence of air in a band of dentinal tubules, such a band appears dark in the section and is called a *dead tract* (Fig. 10–18).

SCLEROTIC (TRANSPARENT) DENTIN. With age, the contents of the dentinal tubules, excluding the odontoblastic processes, may slowly undergo calcification. This takes place especially in the peripheral dentin and in the root dentin. In a ground section of dentin, the organic tubular contents, which are not calcified, deflect light rays passing through the section. This enables us to *see* the tubules and it makes the dentin an opaque tissue.

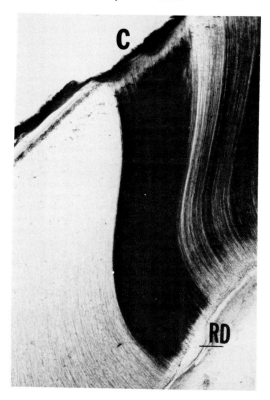

Fig. 10–18. A dead tract in a ground section of a human tooth near the cervix. The S-shaped tubules of the dead tract have filled with air during histologic processing. As a result, they appear dark in ground section. On one end of the dead tract a carious lesion is present (C). On the other end a light patch of reactive dentin (RD) may be seen. The reactive dentin is localized in the area of the insult only. Original magnification × 10.

However, when the contents of the tubules are calcified, the light rays pass relatively straight through the section, without deflection, making it a *transparent* tissue. We call this *transparent* or *sclerotic* dentin. Turnover of the ground substance in such tissue is much more difficult and slower than in normal dentin. For this reason sclerotic dentin may become more brittle with time.

Transparent or sclerotic dentin is also formed adjacent to carious dentin. During the caries attack, the dentin is locally decalcified by the action of the acid produced by the bacteria. The minerals liberated during this decalcification may form new crystals in adjacent dentinal tubules, which may already be empty (a dead tract). The remnants of the tubular contents of such tubules are calcified by the re-crystallizing minerals. Again, when the contents of such tubules become calcified, the tissue in that area becomes transparent.

SELECTED READING LIST

Dental Pulp

Appleton, J., and Williams, M.J.R.: Ultrastructural observations on the calcification of human dental pulp. Calc. Tiss. Res., *11*:222, 1973.

Bernick, S.: Lymphatic vessels of the human dental pulp. J. Dent. Res., *56*:70, 1977.

Fearnhead, R.W.: Innervation of dental tissue. In *Structural and Chemical Organization of Teeth*. Vol. I. Edited by A.E.W. Miles. New York, Academic Press, 1967.

Finn, S.B. (Ed.): *Biology of the Dental Pulp Organ. A Symposium*. Birmingham, University of Alabama, University of Alabama Press, 1968.

Frank, R. M., Wiedemann, P., and Fellinger, E.: Ultrastructure of lymphatic capillaries in the human dental pulp. Cell Tissue Res., *178*:229, 1977.

Gvozdenovic-Sedlecki, S., Qvist, V., and Hansen, H.P.: Histologic variations in the pulp of intact premolars from young individuals. Scand. J. Dent. Res., *81*:433, 1973.

Kukletová, M.: An electron microscopic study of the lymphatic vessels in the dental pulp of the calf. Arch. Oral. Biol., *15*:1117, 1970.

Ogilvie, A.L., and Ingle, J.I.: *An Atlas of Pulpal and Periapical Biology*. Philadelphia, Lea & Febiger, 1965.

Plačková, A., and Vahl, J.: Ultrastructure of mineralizations in the human pulp. Caries Res., *8*:172, 1974.

Rapp, R., El-Labban, N.G., Kramer, I.R.H., and Wood, D.: Ultrastructure of fenestrated capillaries in human dental pulps. Arch. Oral Biol., *22*:317, 1977.

Seltzer, S., and Bender, I.B.: *The Dental Pulp. Biologic Considerations in Dental Procedures*. Philadelphia, J.B. Lippincott Co., 1965.

Siskin, M.: *The Biology of the Human Dental Pulp*. St. Louis, The C.V. Mosby Co., 1973.

Stenvik, A., and Mjör, I.A.: Epithelial remnants and denticle formation in the human dental pulp. Acta Odont. Scand., *28*:721, 1970.

Symons, N.B.B. (Ed.): *Dentine and Pulp*. Edinburgh, E.S. Livingstone Ltd., 1968.

Dentin

Årwill, T., Edwall, L., Lilja, J., Olgart, L., and Svensson, S-E.: Ultrastructure of nerves in the dentinal-pulp border zone after sensory and autonomic nerve transection in the cat. Acta Odont. Scand., *31*:273, 1973.

Bradford, E.W.: Microanatomy and histochemistry of dentin. In *Structural and Chemical Organization of Teeth*. Vol. II. Edited by A.E.W. Miles. New York, Academic Press, 1967.

Brännström, M., and Åström, A.: The hydrodynamics of the dentine. Its possible relationship to dentinal pain. Int. Dent. J., *22*:219, 1972.

Brännström, M., and Garberoglio, R.: The dentinal tubules and the odontoblast processes. A scanning electron microscopic study. Acta Odont. Scand., *30*:291, 1972.

Brännström, M., and Johnson, G.: Effect of various conditioners and cleaning agents on prepared dentin surfaces. A scanning electron microscopic investigation. J. Prosth. Dent., *31*:422, 1974.

Johansen, E.: Ultrastructure of dentine. In *Structural and Chemical Organization of Teeth*. Vol. II. Edited by A.E.W. Miles. New York, Academic Press, 1967.

Johnson, G., and Brännström, M.: The sensitivity of dentin. Changes in relation to conditions at exposed tubule apertures. Acta Odont. Scand., *32*:29, 1974.

Osborn, J.W.: A mechanistic view of dentinogenesis and its relation to the curvatures of the processes of the odontoblasts. Arch. Oral Biol., 12:275, 1967.

Philippas, G.G., and Applebaum, E.: Age factor in secondary dentin formation. J. Dent. Res., 45:778, 1966.

Selvig, K.A.: Ultrastructural changes in human dentine exposed to a weak acid. Arch. Oral Biol., 13:719, 1968.

Shimauchi, K., Yoshie, T., Hasegawa, S., Fujioka, D., Kizu, T., and Ikeda, K.: A scanning electron microscope study of intratubular dentin fibers. J. Nihon Univ. Sch. Dent., 15:113, 1973.

Skinner, H.C.W.: Tetracycline and mineralized tissues. Review and perspectives. Yale Univ. J. Biol. Med., 48:377, 1975.

Symons, N.B.B.: The microanatomy and histochemistry of dentinogenesis. In *Structural and Chemical Organization of Teeth*. Vol I. Edited by A.E.W. Miles. New York, Academic Press, 1967.

Takuma, S.: Ultrastructure of dentinogenesis. In *Structural and Chemical Organization of Teeth*. Vol I. Edited by A.E.W. Miles. New York, Academic Press, 1967.

Chapter **11**

ENAMEL

Enamel covers the anatomical crowns of the teeth. It is the hardest tissue found in the human body. This hardness results from its high degree of calcification. The mineral hydroxyapatite makes up 95% of the total weight of enamel, compared with 70% of the total weight in dentin and 45% of the total weight in bone.

A small amount of epithelially produced enamel matrix is present in mature enamel, only about 1% of the total weight. Water is responsible for the remaining 4%. If the mineral is removed from enamel by decalcification, the remaining enamel matrix is so delicate that it disintegrates and leaves an empty space behind in decalcified sections of a tooth. Because of this property, enamel is studied with the light microscope almost exclusively in ground sections.

If any enamel matrix remains in a routinely decalcified section, you may be assured that this matrix was incompletely calcified before the tooth was placed in the fixating agent. This may be the case in developing teeth, in which part of the enamel matrix has not yet been broken down and resorbed during enamel maturation. In mature teeth, the presence of enamel matrix in a histologic section indicates that a disturbance occurred during enamel maturation.

One may become acquainted with the structure of enamel by using an old method to study it:

Place a newly extracted tooth in 12 ml of a 10% HCl solution. At the end of 30 hours in this acid, the enamel is partially decalcified and quite soft. Remove a small portion of this softened tissue with a needle or a brush and place it on a microscopic glass slide. Now carefully tease out this mass thinly with fine needles. Place a drop of saline solution on this preparation and cover it with a small cover glass. The preparation may be stained by allowing a histologic stain to run beneath the cover glass by capillary action.

When you study this material with the light microscope, you will notice that the enamel has been separated into what seem to be fine fibers. Actually, these are the cores of the structural units of the tissue enamel. The units of enamel, *enamel prisms* or *rods,* are highly calcified rods, with little enamel matrix, separated from each other by thin, noncalcified sheaths of enamel matrix, the *prism sheaths.*

CLINICALLY IMPORTANT FEATURES
OF ENAMEL

GROOVES OR FISSURES IN THE OCCLUSAL SURFACES OF MOLARS AND PREMOLARS. During tooth development, the enamel-forming cells, the ameloblasts, move from the dentino-enamel junction outward. This means that these cells move from a smaller area to a larger one, when they are located on one of the tooth's *convex* surfaces. However, the areas between adjacent cusps of molars and premolars are *concave,* and the ameloblasts on these surfaces have the same problems as do the odontoblasts during dentin production: they soon suffer from crowding.

In the deeper parts of these concave surfaces, ameloblasts occasionally "back into each other." These cells become compressed, and they are cut off from their sources of nutrition. The result is cell death of the affected ameloblasts and incomplete maturation of the enamel matrix, which is produced by these cells.

This leads to the presence of a "weak spot" in the tooth's defense against caries. The incompletely calcified areas are readily attacked by caries. The situation is further complicated by the fact that the perished ameloblasts leave a deep, thin groove (thinner than the dental probe in most cases) in the occlusal surface. Food remnants and bacteria are easily caught and retained in such grooves, and they are hard to remove, even with careful toothbrushing (Fig. 11–1).

These grooves and fissures are real trouble spots, where caries can easily occur. Some prevention of these problems may result from the application of a protective coating or a *sealant,* which covers the grooves of the occlusal surfaces for some time.

ORIENTATION OF ENAMEL PRISMS. The ultimate success of a restoration in a tooth depends to a large extent on a good cavity preparation. For a good cavity preparation it is critically important to know the course of enamel prisms.

$\rightarrow$

Fig. 11–1.   A, *An x-ray of a ground section through a premolar shows the presence of a deep occlusal fissure* (arrow). *The entrance to this fissure is too narrow for a dental probe. The enamel around the deep end of the fissure is incompletely calcified.* × 1. B, *The contents of a fissure in a decalcified section of the tooth shown in* A. *What looked like an empty groove on the x-ray is in fact filled with organic debris and bacteria* (arrow). *Some partially calcified enamel matrix is visible as well. Original magnification* × 5.

As a rule, all enamel prisms run from the dentino-enamel junction to the outer enamel surface, across the entire width of the enamel. This means that the *length* of an enamel prism depends on its location. Near the cusps, or near the incisal edges, the prisms are long (3 to 4 mm); near the cervix of the tooth, where the enamel is knife-edged, the prisms are almost negligible in length.

The average *width* of an enamel prism is about 4 μm, but this width varies; near the dentino-enamel junction the prisms are narrower and near the outer enamel surface they are wider. As we shall see, even in one cross section, an enamel prism is not of even width.

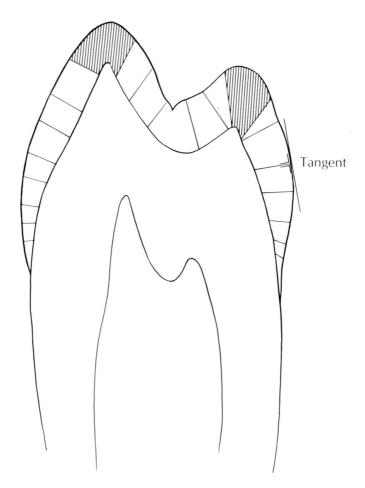

Tangent

Fig. 11–2. *Diagram indicating the general orientations of enamel prisms as lines within the enamel cap. Generally, all prisms run from the dentino-enamel junction perpendicularly to the tangent of the enamel surface. The areas of gnarled enamel at the cusps, where enamel prisms have a more complicated course, are hatched.*

As an easy rule of thumb, it should be remembered that enamel prisms run toward the outer enamel surface, like the spokes in a wheel, *perpendicular* to the outer surface, or more precisely, to its tangents. Near the cervix, the prisms are oriented somewhat more apically. Most prisms are *wavy* near the dentino-enamel junction, but they are relatively straight near the enamel surface (Fig. 11–2).

The course of the enamel prisms is complicated in the enamel of a cusp or incisal edge. Here the prisms are twisted around each other, and when studied in a ground section, single prisms are hard to follow from the dentino-enamel junction to the outer surface. Such enamel is called *gnarled enamel*.

Prisms are clinically important because isolated enamel prisms, or parts of enamel prisms, are extremely brittle and break easily. The strength of intact enamel is attributable, to a great degree, to its support by the underlying dentin. When cutting through enamel during a cavity preparation, it is essential to *leave no enamel prisms unsupported by dentin*. If a prism, or part of a prism, is undercut at the edge of a cavity preparation, it will break off easily, making the margin of the restoration defective and leaky.

The designs of all types of cavity preparations take the course of the enamel prisms into account. Since it is nearly impossible to avoid undercut enamel prisms in gnarled enamel at a cusp or incisal edge, the margins of restorations are usually placed in non-gnarled enamel.

DIFFERENTIAL ETCHING PATTERNS IN ENAMEL. In recent years, sealants have been introduced. Application of such mate-

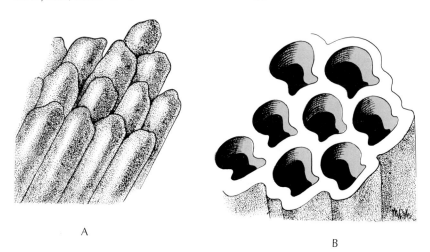

A

B

Fig. 11–3. Diagram showing, in strong magnification and with exaggeration, the effects of acid etching on enamel. The acid may preferentially attack, to a certain depth, the prism sheaths and peripheries, leaving the prism cores behind, A. Or, the prism cores may be etched away to a certain depth, leaving a honeycomb of prism peripheries and sheaths behind, B.

Fig. 11–4. Actual appearance of etched enamel surfaces, as seen with the scanning electron microscope. A, Survey of an etched enamel surface. The etching pattern in the top half of the photograph differs from the pattern in the bottom half. Original magnification ×1000. B, Detail from the bottom half of the area shown in A. In this part of the etched surface, the prism cores have been left preferentially. Most etching has occurred in the horseshoe-shaped depressions, which correspond with the prism sheaths around the "heads" of the enamel prisms (this chapter). Original magnification × 5000.

Fig. 11–4. (Cont'd)   C, Detail from the top half of the area shown in A. In this part of the etched surface, the prism peripheries have been left preferentially, resulting in a rough, honeycomb-like pattern. Original magnification × 5000. (Courtesy Dr. A.J. Gwinnett.)

rials on tooth surfaces protects these surfaces against caries for a certain period of time. Comparable materials have been introduced that attach orthodontic brackets directly to tooth surfaces without the use of metal bands (direct bonding technique).

If such materials would be applied directly to untreated enamel, they would detach easily, since they are unable to hold onto the smooth enamel surface. The enamel surface has to be roughened first, and this is done by *etching* it for a brief period of time. The concept of etching depends on the fact that enamel consists of prisms and prism sheaths, with different compositions.

Etching is done by the application of an acid to the tooth surface. The acid penetrates for a short distance (about 30 μm) into the enamel. Initially, the acid probably moves more easily through the uncalcified prism sheaths, attacking the mineral at the peripheries of the prisms and leaving the prism cores behind. This gives the treated enamel surface a rougher texture.

In some areas the prism sheaths seem to be relatively impermeable to the acid. Here the acid attacks the prism cores preferentially, leaving a honeycomb-like pattern of prism sheaths behind. This too makes the enamel surface rougher. It makes, therefore, no difference which part of the enamel tissue is etched away, as long as there is a differential etching pattern, which leaves the surface of the enamel rougher (Figs. 11–3 and 11–4).

The sealants and bonding materials form little spurs in the spaces where the enamel has been etched away. Such spurs hold these materials firmly attached to the tooth surface.

In some teeth, especially the newly emerged primary teeth, the outer layer of enamel has no prism structure. This layer may be 100 to 150 μm thick, and it is composed of evenly calcified enamel matrix *(prismless layer)*.

Etching of such a homogeneous layer will not appreciably roughen the enamel surface, since most etching procedures depend on the different compositions of prisms and prism sheaths and do not affect the enamel to a level deeper than 30 μm. The etching and the subsequent attachment of sealants and bonding materials may be less successful in such cases.

ENAMEL PRISMS AND PRISM SHEATHS

You have learned already that the structural units of enamel are *enamel prisms:* rod-like structures running from the dentino-enamel junction to the outer enamel surface. Their lengths are determined by the local enamel thickness, while their *average* diameters are 4 μm. Neighboring enamel prisms are separated from each other by 0.1- to 0.2-μm-wide *prism sheaths.*

The distinction between enamel prisms and prism sheaths is based primarily on their relative amounts of enamel matrix and their relative degrees of calcification. In the prisms the hydroxyapatite occupies nearly all available space, leaving little for the enamel matrix components. In contrast, the prism sheaths consist almost exclusively of enamel matrix, with little or no hydroxyapatite present.

$\rightarrow$

Fig. 11–5. A, *Idealized cross sections through enamel prisms, showing the keyhole-shaped outlines of the individual prisms. The prisms are stacked together in an intricate, interlocking pattern.* B, *Three-dimensional diagram of an enamel prism. The prism runs from left to right, from the dentino-enamel junction to the outer enamel surface. A section is left out, to indicate that the prism at this magnification would be considerably longer than the page. The rounded head of the enamel prism faces the cuspal/incisal region of the tooth, while the thin tail region faces the cervix of the tooth. Inside the prism, the orientation of the long, thin, needle-like hydroxyapatite crystallites is indicated. In the head region of the prism the crystallites run parallel to the long axis of the prism. In the tail region they run perpendicular to the long axis of the prism.* C, *The orientation of the hydroxyapatite crystallites is shown in this diagram of a cross section through several enamel prisms. In the head regions the hydroxyapatite crystallites are cut transversely, while in the tail regions the crystallites are cut along their lengths.*

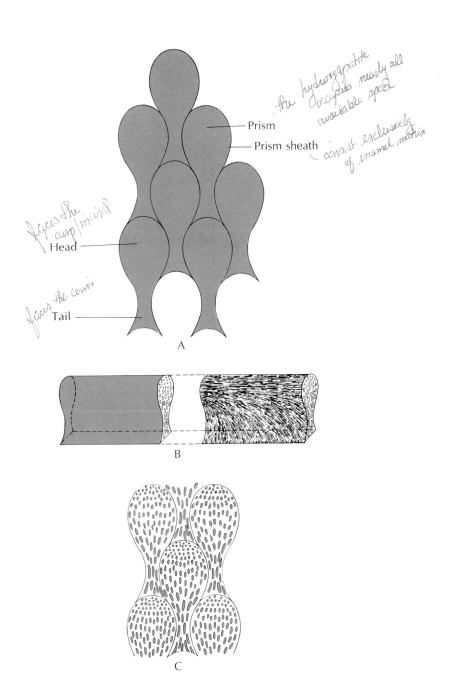

A

Prism

Prism sheath

Head

Tail

the hydroxyapatite occupies nearly all available space

consist exclusively of enamel matrix

faces the cusp/incisal

faces the cervix

B

C

In cross section the prisms in human enamel most frequently have a keyhole shape. The rounded heads of these keyholes are pointed toward the occlusal/incisal ends of the teeth, while their tails are pointed cervically.

The rows of prisms are stacked fairly neatly, with the tails of one prism layer interlocked with the rounded heads of a second layer of prisms, which is located below the first layer, and touching the tops of the rounded heads of a third prism layer, which is located below the second one (Fig. 11–5, A). The prism sheaths are distinctly visible around the rounded heads of the prisms, but they become blurred, or even absent, around the thinner tails of the prisms.

The small crystals of the mineral salt *(hydroxyapatite crystallites)* in enamel are unusual in that they are about 4 times larger, in all dimensions, than the hydroxyapatite crystallites in bone, dentin or cementum. These hydroxyapatite crystallites run within each enamel prism with their *long axes parallel* to the long axis of the prism in the rounded *head* area, but *perpendicular* to the long axis of the prism in the *tail* area (Fig. 11–5, B, C). In the area between the head and the tail of one enamel prism, there is a gradual change in the orientation of the hydroxyapatite crystallites.

Prism sheaths are most pronounced where they separate 2 groups of hydroxyapatite crystallites, running at right angles to each other: one group in the top of the rounded head of one prism and the other group in the bottom of the tail of the prism directly above the first one.

DEVELOPMENT OF ENAMEL PRISMS. The average diameter of an enamel-producing cell (ameloblast) is about 4 μm, comparable to the average diameter of an enamel prism. Although there are, during development, as many ameloblasts as there are enamel prisms in the fully formed tooth, each enamel prism is *not* produced by one single ameloblast. This point may be understood by superimposing the cross-sectional outlines of a sheet of ameloblasts over the cross-sectional outlines of the enamel prisms produced by these ameloblasts. There is an *uneven overlap.*

The ameloblasts are hexagonal in cross section. (This provides a highly efficient packing system, comparable to the structure of a honeycomb.) Most enamel prisms are keyhole-shaped in cross section. The rounded head of an enamel prism is produced by one ameloblast, but its tail is produced by contributions of 3 adjacent ameloblasts (Fig. 11–6).

The specific shape of an enamel prism and the peculiar relationship between prism and ameloblasts are the result of the particular *shape* of the *Tomes' process* of a *human ameloblast.* As we saw before, the Tomes' process is shovel-shaped, with a wide, hexagonal base and a thin, horseshoe-shaped, knife-edge tip (Fig. 11–7).

During enamel matrix formation, hydroxyapatite crystallites are deposited in this matrix, with their long axes perpendicular to the

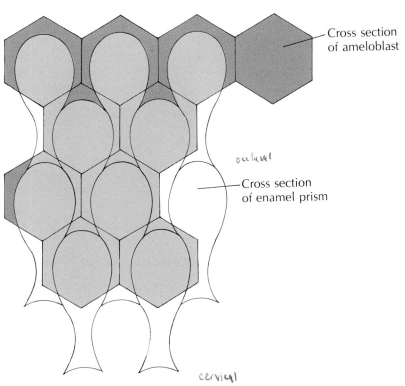

Cross section
of ameloblast

occlusal

Cross section
of enamel prism

cervical

Fig. 11–6. *The cross sectional, hexagonal outlines of ameloblasts are superimposed over the cross sectional, keyhole-shaped outlines of the enamel prisms produced by the ameloblasts. Notice that each ameloblast contributes to the formation of 4 enamel prisms, while each enamel prism is formed by contributions from 4 ameloblasts.*

cell membrane of the Tomes' process. There is an abrupt change in the orientation of the crystallites, where there is an abrupt change in the orientation of the cell membrane of the Tomes' process: at its thin, horseshoe-shaped edge. As the result of this abrupt change in the crystallite orientation, an interface without crystallites remains between the 2 groups of crystallites. This interface is the future prism sheath (Fig. 11–8).

During maturation (further calcification) of the enamel matrix, the existing crystallites increase in thickness and in width, but not in length or in number. Thus, the original width of the areas without crystallites, the prism sheaths, remains about the same, with only a minimal reduction compared with its original dimensions.

The knife edge of the Tomes' process is the only really sharp edge of this process, producing a distinct prism sheath around the rounded head of the enamel prism. Elsewhere, the sheath becomes

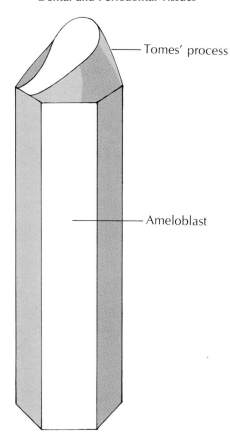

Fig. 11–7. Somewhat simplified, diagrammatic representation of an ameloblast in 3 dimensions. The ameloblast has a tall, columnar cell body, hexagonal in cross section. At its secretory end, a shovel-shaped Tomes' process is present with a thin, horseshoe-shaped, knife-edge tip. The light area of the Tomes' process in this diagram is slightly concave.

blurred or even absent. There is no difference in orientation between the cell membranes of adjacent Tomes' processes. Therefore it is possible for more than one ameloblast to contribute to one enamel prism, without the formation of seams, to delineate the contributions of the 4 different cells.

The gradual slope of the Tomes' process is responsible for the deposition of hydroxyapatite crystallites, which gradually change their orientation in the zone between the rounded head and the tail of the enamel prism.

Finally, areas of *prismless enamel* are found frequently near the dentino-enamel junction and near the outer surface of the enamel. Their presence may be explained by the *absence* of distinct Tomes'

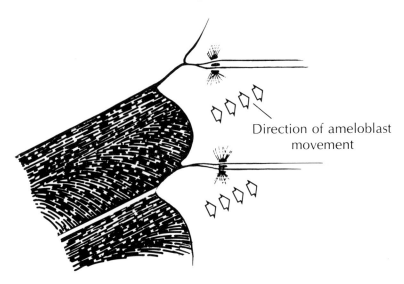

Direction of ameloblast
movement

Fig. 11–8. *Illustration of the formation of enamel prisms, during enamel deposition by the ameloblasts. The ameloblasts are located to the right. They move backward, in the direction indicated by the arrows, during their secretory activities. In the newly deposited enamel matrix, the hydroxyapatite crystallites are oriented perpendicular to the membrane of the Tomes' process. Where the process makes its sharp knife-edge (see Fig. 11–7), the crystallites run at right angles to each other. Between these 2 groups of crystallites, the prism sheath is located. It is an area of enamel matrix with few, if any, crystallites between 2 groups of crystallites running at right angles to each other.*

processes at the times these layers of enamel were deposited. Near the dentino-enamel junction, the ameloblasts may not immediately form a Tomes' process after they have differentiated and have begun depositing enamel matrix. At or near the completion of their secretory activities, the ameloblasts lose their Tomes' processes again. A layer of ameloblasts without Tomes' processes forms a smooth, straight surface. All hydroxyapatite crystallites are deposited perpendicular to this surface and parallel to each other. No prisms or prism sheaths are formed in this way.

   CURVATURES OF ENAMEL PRISMS. In the introduction of this chapter we noted that enamel prisms do not run entirely straight from the dentino-enamel junction to the outer enamel surface.

   The prisms are curved predominantly in the *inner third* of the thickness of enamel (nearest the dentino-enamel junction). These curves can be demonstrated clearly on an extracted tooth which has been broken in half *lengthwise*. Near the dentino-enamel junction the fracture surface is not flat, but wavy. Since these waves are visible with the unaided eye, each wave must consist of *groups* of enamel prisms, not single ones.

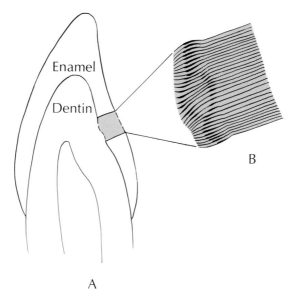

B

A

Fig. 11-9. Diagram of a tooth, broken in half lengthwise. The fracture surface is not smooth, but, as shown in insert B, the surface is very wavy near the dentino-enamel junction. Groups of prisms curve upward above the general plane of the fracture surface, or downward, below this plane. In this picture 2 groups of upward curving prisms are shown, on either side of a group of downward curving prisms, B. In the transition areas, between upward and downward curving prisms, groups of prisms run more or less within the general plane of the fracture surface. Similarly, in the outer two thirds of the enamel width, all prisms run more or less smoothly within this plane.

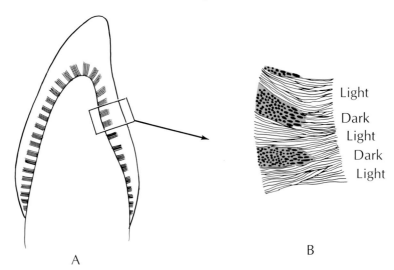

Light
Dark
Light
Dark
Light

B

A

Fig. 11-10. In a smoothly ground section of a tooth, the surface of the section is no longer wavy, as it is in a fractured tooth. Groups of prisms, curving either upward or downward, relative to the fracture plane, are both partially cross sectioned, near the dentino-enamel junction, B. Only in the outer enamel and in the transitional regions, between upward and downward curving groups of prisms, the prisms are cut lengthwise. As a result, when a longitudinal ground section is viewed with incident light (not light transmitted through the section), the cross sectioned enamel prisms appear dark in the reflected light, while the longitudinally sectioned prisms appear light.

These waves are produced by groups of enamel prisms curving *above* the level of the fracture plane, *alternating* with groups of prisms that curve *below* the level of the fracture plane. Thus, the first group makes convexities and the second group makes concavities relative to the fracture plane of the tooth. Between the 2 groups another group of prisms runs more or less straight, at the *level* of the fracture plane (Fig. 11–9).

If one were to make a ground section of a tooth, the last group of prisms would be cut along the long axes of these prisms in the section. The other 2 groups would be cut obliquely or in cross section. The prisms that curved above the fracture plane would first run out of this section toward the viewer and then back into the section, away from the viewer, when the enamel is scanned from the dentino-enamel junction toward the outer surface. The prisms that curved below the fracture plane would first run into the section and later out of the section, under the same conditions (Fig. 11–10).

Such alternately longitudinally and transversely sectioned groups of enamel prisms are called *Hunter-Schreger bands*. These bands are only visible if a tooth is sectioned along its longitudinal axis,

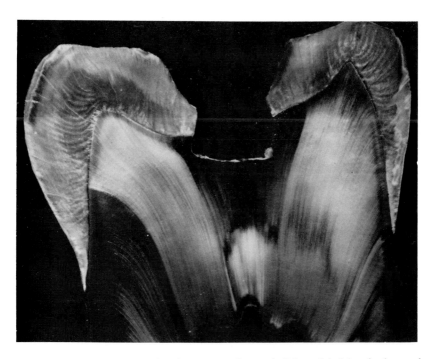

Fig. 11–11. Hunter-Schreger bands appear as alternately light and dark bands of enamel prisms, running from the dentino-enamel junction outwards to about one half the width of the enamel cap, in a longitudinal ground section of a human molar, viewed with incident and reflected light. Original magnification × 2.

because the waves of the enamel prisms are oriented predominantly in a horizontal plane (Fig. 11–11).

OTHER FEATURES OF ENAMEL

We have purposely stressed the *clinical* importance of understanding the differences in composition between enamel prisms and prism sheaths and the course of the enamel prisms.

However, since enamel is a complicated tissue, with several additional points of interest, some of these will be discussed briefly.

Enamel, once deposited, is not remodeled. Since enamel-forming cells, or ameloblasts, are lost shortly after the emergence of the tooth in the oral cavity, no additional enamel is formed after this event. Thus, the crown of a tooth does *not* increase further in size, and enamel is incapable of repair. Any imperfections in the enamel, produced during enamel formation, remain present in this tissue throughout the functional life of the tooth.

CROSS-STRIATIONS OF ENAMEL PRISMS. In a ground section of enamel, especially after light decalcification, alternately light and dark cross striations are visible in the enamel prisms. These cross striations are 4 to 8 μm apart and they are comparable with the imbrication lines (von Ebner) in the dentin, in that they are

Fig. 11–12. Enamel prisms, running from left to right, with vertical cross striations (arrows). The large, dark bands, running obliquely across the photograph, are incremental lines (Retzius). Notice that the cross striations are more distinct in these incremental lines. In a longitudinal section of a tooth, the incremental lines run characteristically at an angle to both the enamel prisms and the cross striations. Original magnification × 125.

probably produced as the result of differences in the enamel deposition during day- and nighttime (Fig. 11–12).

The enamel matrix in the light striations may differ somewhat from the matrix in the dark striations; the light striations may be a little better calcified than the dark striations. In addition, the individual enamel prisms have alternate constrictions and bulges along their length, respectively corresponding to the dark and the light cross striations.

INCREMENTAL LINES (RETZIUS). If, during enamel formation, the organism is under some stress (disease, birth), the enamel deposited at that time may show some irregularities in its calcification and a disruption of the course of the enamel prisms, producing *incremental lines* (Fig. 11–13).

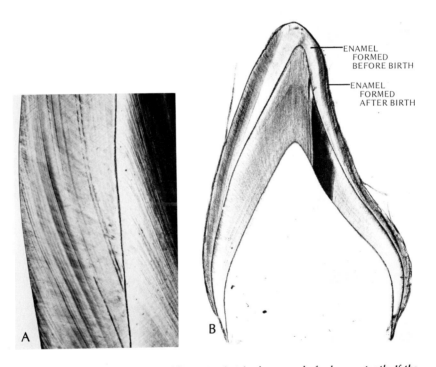

ENAMEL
FORMED
BEFORE BIRTH

ENAMEL
FORMED
AFTER BIRTH

A   B

Fig. 11–13. **A,** *Dark, incremental lines (Retzius) in the enamel of a human tooth. If the tooth is cut lengthwise, as is the case in this ground section, the incremental lines run from the dentino-enamel junction obliquely outward, in the direction of incisal edge or cusps (located at the top of the picture). In a cross section through a tooth, the incremental lines run parallel with the dentino-enamel junction and with the outer enamel surface. Original magnification* × *12.5.* **B,** *Ground section of the anatomical crown of a primary incisor tooth. The enamel, formed before birth, is light, better calcified than the enamel formed after birth. Several incremental lines are present in the darker postnatal enamel. Notice also the fainter corresponding contour lines (Owen) in the dentin. Original magnification* × *2.*

In ground sections, such incremental lines, which correspond with the contour lines (Owen) in the dentin, usually appear dark as the result of their relatively lesser degree of calcification and a correspondingly larger amount of enamel matrix. Frequently, adjacent to such a dark line, a lighter line of well-calcified enamel may be present (perhaps better calcified in reaction to the incomplete calcification of the preceding layer ?).

The course of the enamel prisms is usually disturbed in an incremental line. The prisms may have a zig-zag orientation, and in some cases they may even lose their sharp distinction completely and prismless enamel may locally replace them.

In all teeth of the primary dentition and in the first molars of the secondary dentition, an extra sharp incremental line may be present, identified as a neonatal line. Occasionally, the line is not clear, but the differences between enamel formed prenatally and enamel formed postnatally may be striking. Usually the prenatally formed enamel is regular and highly calcified, whereas the postnatally formed enamel is somewhat irregular and less calcified. However, in some teeth this may be reversed. Clearly, it depends on the quality of intrauterine life, compared with the quality of life after birth, which may be variable for different individuals.

Near the cervix of the tooth, large numbers of regularly spaced incremental lines may be found in the enamel. Their regular spacing seems to suggest that something other than disease may be involved in the production of those lines. Because of the pattern of deposition of enamel, the lines in the cervical area run obliquely from the dentino-enamel junction to the outside surface of the enamel. External manifestations of these lines are visible as linear dips (perikymata), running all around the enamel surface in newly erupted teeth. Except in protected areas, these perikymata are rapidly worn down during the function of the teeth.

In contrast with the situation in dentin, the antibiotic tetracycline does not form distinct incremental lines in enamel, owing to the differences in the nature of enamel and dentin matrices and the differences in the way these matrices calcify. In high doses tetracycline may temporarily disturb the ameloblasts, and this may lead to defects in the enamel being formed at that time. Such defects may take up some of the tetracycline.

DENTINO-ENAMEL JUNCTION AND ENAMEL SPINDLES. The dentino-enamel junction is frequently scalloped rather than smooth. The rounded, convex sides of such a scalloped surface are always facing the dentin, while the concavities are facing the enamel. It is not clear precisely what causes this scalloping. It must happen during tooth development, in the brief period between the breakdown of the basal lamina, a straight and smooth structure separating odontoblasts from preameloblasts, and the first deposition of dentin and enamel. Once the first layers of dentin and

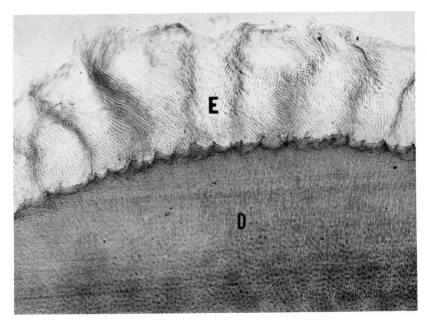

Fig. 11–14. Scalloped dentino-enamel junction in a decalcified cross section of a develop-ing tooth. The not yet fully calcified enamel matrix (E) is preserved, showing the wavy course of the enamel prisms, in different directions at different vertical levels. The concavities of the dentino-enamel junction face the enamel, while the rounded, convex sides face the dentin (D). Notice the relative proportions of the enamel prism diameters and the sizes of the concavities of the dentino-enamel junction. Original magnification × 125.

enamel are laid down, these 2 hard tissues preserve the existing morphology of the dentino-enamel junction (Fig. 11–14).

The scalloping of the dentino-enamel junction takes place at a time when a great deal of motion is taking place in this region. You will remember that, following the breakdown of the basal lamina, cell processes of both odontoblasts and preameloblasts extend across this former border. They make contact with each other, which leads to the differentiation of ameloblasts and the start of enamel production.

The processes themselves are not responsible for the scalloping of the junction. The concavities of this scalloped surface are broad, corresponding to a large number of enamel prisms and thus, at an earlier time, to large numbers of odontoblasts and ameloblasts.

Some of the odontoblastic processes are not withdrawn rapidly enough, following their interactions with the preameloblastic cell processes. The first deposited enamel surrounds such processes, leaving a few small defects in the enamel, in the form of short, blind-ending tubules. Since they are frequently spindle-shaped, these structures are called *spindles*.

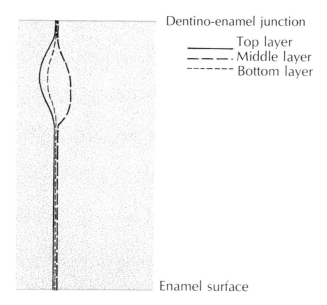

Dentino-enamel junction

——————— Top layer
— — — —. Middle layer
------- Bottom layer

Enamel surface

Fig. 11–15.   Diagram of enamel in a thick cross section of a tooth. The dentino-enamel junction is shown at the top, while the outer enamel surface is shown at the bottom of the figure. The orientations of enamel prisms at 3 vertical levels (layers) of the thick ground section are shown. The prisms curve, in a horizontal plane, especially near the dentino-enamel junction (the same curves produce the wavy fracture surface, shown in Fig. 11–9). At different vertical levels, the prisms curve in different directions. All prisms straighten out in the outer enamel.

They are recognizable as short extensions of some of the dentinal tubules, crossing the dentino-enamel junction into the enamel. Their course is independent of the course of the enamel prisms. Since the dentinal tubules in mature dentin no longer contain part of the odontoblastic processes near the dentino-enamel junction, the spindles also are most likely to be empty, apart from some tissue fluid.

The scalloping of the dentino-enamel junction is most pronounced near the tips of cusps and incisal edges. Similarly, the largest numbers of spindles are found in these regions. Toward the cervix of the tooth the dentino-enamel junction becomes straight, and the dentino-cementum junction in the root similarly continues in straight fashion.

TUFTS AND LAMELLAE. Tufts and lamellae are normal features in enamel, consisting of characteristically shaped defects of calcification.

Tufts are found in the inner third layer of enamel, the same layer in which the course of the enamel prisms is curved. Tufts consist of noncalcified parts of enamel prisms, appearing dark in ground sections. In a horizontal ground section, through the crown of a tooth, tufts resemble bundles of grass. Each "leaf" in such a bundle is located at a different vertical level within the section. The leaves all originate from one vertical line along the dentino-enamel junction, and since a vertical line in a horizontal projection is represented by a point, all leaves of the tuft seem to originate at that same point in a horizontal section.

The appearance of a bundle of grass leaves, all fanning out in different directions, is caused by the fact that enamel prisms at different vertical levels *curve* in different directions (see the section on Hunter-Schreger bands in this chapter). The uncalcified parts of the prisms follow the same course as the surrounding calcified prisms at their particular vertical level (Fig. 11–15).

When you are viewing a tuft with the microscope, notice that you are able to focus on only one vertical level of the ground section at any time. Thus, only the "leaf of grass" of the tuft, which is located in that particular level, will be clearly in focus. The other leaves of the tuft are less clear and out of focus (Fig. 11–16).

Focusing up and down with the microscope will enable you to bring different levels of the tuft in focus consecutively, giving you a three-dimensional appreciation of this structure.

It is not clear what causes the formation of tufts. The suggestion has been made that, within certain tension planes, internal stress in the developing tissue prevents parts of prisms from calcification. What produces this internal stress has not been resolved. Perhaps the ameloblasts themselves, moving backward in different directions, at different vertical levels (remember the different curvatures of the enamel prisms), produce these tension planes.

Lamellae also originate at the dentino-enamel junction, but these structures run across the entire width of the enamel. Lamellae are uncalcified vertical sheets of organic material. They may have the same height as the anatomical crown, but more frequently they are about half as high, running from the cervix of the tooth occlusally (Fig. 11–17).

Lamellae may form in at least 3 different ways, producing noncalcified organic sheets of different compositions.

1. *LAMELLAE CONSISTING OF UNCALCIFIED ENAMEL MATRIX.* These lamellae are similar to tufts in appearance and in the way they form. However, while tufts are limited to the inner third of the enamel, lamellae run through the entire enamel width. This type of lamella develops while enamel is being deposited by the ameloblasts. They probably represent a tension plane in which entire prisms, as well as large parts of prisms, failed to calcify.

Fig. 11–16. *Tufts in a horizontal ground section of a human tooth. The dark tufts run from the dentino-enamel junction to approximately one-third of the enamel width. A, B and C show different planes of focus (which means different vertical levels) of the same section. Different "leaves" of each tuft are in focus in the different photographs, illustrating the different courses of enamel prisms in these different vertical levels. Original magnification × 50.*

Fig. 11–17. A, Spindles (arrows) in a ground section of the cuspal region of a molar tooth. In such regions spindles are particularly abundant. Notice the different shapes of the spindles. All are blind-ending continuations of dentinal tubules across the dentino-enamel junction. Some, however, are just simple extensions, while others have enlarged, club-shaped ends. Original magnification × 50. B, A lamella (asterisk), several tufts and a spindle in a horizontal ground section through a human tooth. Compare the different dimensions and shapes of these 3 structures. The lamella extends all the way across the enamel width. The tufts do not extend beyond one-third of the enamel width. The spindle is only visible in C (arrow). Two dark incremental lines (Retzius) are visible (IL), running parallel to the dentino-enamel junction and to the enamel surface. Original magnification B, × 12.5; Insert, × 50.

2. *LAMELLAE CONSISTING OF CELLULAR DEBRIS OF THE ENAMEL ORGAN.* During tooth development, and prior to the emergence of the tooth into the oral cavity, the developing, or just completed, enamel may fracture. What causes such fractures is not clear at this time, but we know that they do occur. The fracture becomes filled with cells of the enamel organ and other organic matter. The result is an organic sheet, or lamella, interrupting the continuity of the calcified enamel.

The preceding 2 types of lamellae were lamellae formed *during tooth development*. The third type of lamella is produced *after* the *eruption* of the tooth.

3. *LAMELLAE CONSISTING OF ORGANIC DEBRIS FROM THE ORAL CAVITY.* Following the eruption of the tooth, its enamel cap may suffer fractures. These fractures become filled with salivary proteins and cellular debris from the oral cavity, which form the organic substance of this type of lamellae. These lamellae may become more frequent with age, because of the possibility of fractures that may occur as the result of uneven loading of the teeth during function.

SELECTED READING LIST

Boyde, A.: The structure of developing mammalian dental enamel. In *Tooth Enamel.* Edited by M.V. Stack and R.W. Fearnhead. Bristol, John Wright and Sons, 1965.

Crabb, H.S.M., and Darling, A.I.: *The Pattern of Progressive Mineralization of Human Dental Enamel.* New York, Pergamon Press, 1962.

Fearnhead, R.W., and Stack, M.V. (Editors): *Tooth Enamel* II. Bristol, John Wright and Sons, 1971.

Frank, R.M., and Nalbandian, J.: Ultrastructure of amelogenesis. In *Structural and Chemical Organization of Teeth.* Vol. I. Edited by A.E.W. Miles. New York, Academic Press, 1967.

Garant, P.R., and Nalbandian, J.: Observations on the ultrastructure of ameloblasts with special reference to the Golgi complex and related components. J. Ultrastructure Res., 23:427, 1968.

Gustafson, A-G.: A morphologic investigation of certain variations in the structure and mineralisation of human dental enamel. Odont. Tidsk., 67:361, 1959.

Gustafson, G., and Gustafson, A-G.: Microanatomy and histochemistry of enamel. In *Structural and Chemical Organization of Teeth.* Vol. II. Edited by A.E.W. Miles. New York, Academic Press, 1967.

Gwinnett, A.J.: The ultrastructure of the "prismless" enamel of the deciduous teeth. Arch. Oral Biol., 11:1109, 1966.

Gwinnett, A.J.: The ultrastructure of the "prismless" enamel of permanent human teeth. Arch. Oral Biol., 12:381, 1967.

Gwinnett, A.J.: Histologic changes in human enamel following treatment with acidic adhesive conditioning agents. Arch. Oral Biol., 16:731, 1971.

Gwinnett, A.J.: Structural changes in enamel and dentin of fractured anterior teeth after acid conditioning in vitro. JADA, 86:117, 1973.

Helmcke, J-G.: Ultrastructure of enamel. In *Structural and Chemical Organization of Teeth.* Volume II. Edited by A.E.W. Miles. New York, Academic Press, 1967.

Hodson, J.J.: An investigation into the microscopic structure of the common forms of enamel lamellae with special reference to their origin and contents. Oral Surg. Oral Med. Oral Path., 6:305, 1953.

Marshall, G.W., Olson, L.M., and Lee, C.V.: SEM investigation of the variability of enamel surfaces after stimulated clinical acid etching for pit and fissure sealants. J. Dent. Res., *54*:1222, 1975.

Meckel, A.H.: Structure of mature human dental enamel as observed by electron microscopy. Arch. Oral Biol., *10*:775, 1965.

Meckel, A.H., Griebstein, W.J., and Neal, R.J.: Ultrastructure of fully calcified human dental enamel. In *Tooth Enamel.* Edited by M.V. Stack and R.W. Fearnhead. Bristol, John Wright and Sons, 1965.

Osborn, J.W.: The three dimensional morphology of the tufts in human enamel. Acta Anat., *73*:481, 1969.

Osborn, J.W.: Variations in structure and development of enamel. Oral Sciences Reviews, *3*:3, 1973.

Reith, E.J.: The ultrastructure of ameloblasts during matrix formation and the maturation of enamel. J. Biophys., *9*:825, 1961.

Reith, E.J.: The ultrastructure of ameloblasts during early stages of maturation of enamel. J. Cell Biol., *18*:691, 1963.

Rönnholm, E.: An electron microscopic study of the amelogenesis in human teeth. I. The fine structure of the ameloblasts. J. Ultrastructure Res., *6*:229, 1962.

Rönnholm, E.: An electron microscopic study of the amelogenesis in human teeth. II. The development of the enamel crystallites. J. Ultrastructure Res., *6*:249, 1962.

Rönnholm, E.: The structure of the organic stroma of human enamel during amelogenesis. J. Ultrastructure Res., *6*:368, 1962.

Stack, M.V., and Fearnhead, R.W. (Editors): *Tooth Enamel.* Bristol, John Wright and Sons, 1965.

Tyler, J.E.: A scanning electron microscopic study of factors influencing etch patterns of human enamel. Arch. Oral Biol., *21*:765, 1976.

Chapter 12

CEMENTUM AND ALVEOLAR BONE

Cementum and alveolar bone are 2 of the 3 tissues that are responsible for the attachment of the teeth to the bones of the jaws. Cementum covers the dentin of the anatomical root. Alveolar bone is part of the bones of the jaws. The third tissue is the periodontal ligament. It is located between cementum and alveolar bone and it is the topic of the next chapter.

Cementum, periodontal ligament and the inner layer of alveolar bone of the tooth socket are formed during development by cells of the dental sac. These in turn are derived from neural crest cells.

Clinically, both cementum and alveolar bone are needed for the attachment of a functioning tooth, somewhat like the 2 towers of a suspension bridge. If one of the two is missing, the bridge cannot exist.

If *cementum* is not present, as is the case when the root of a primary tooth is resorbed during the eruption of its secondary successor, the tooth becomes loose. Fortunately, most of the time the resorption of cementum is a localized process, so that some surfaces of the root remain covered with cementum, enabling the tooth to continue functioning. During periods of repair, when a small amount of cementum temporarily fills in some of the resorption cavities, the tooth becomes more firmly fixed. This lasts until the next wave of resorptions.

If *alveolar bone* is absent, as in cases of severe periodontal disease, the teeth become loose and useless for chewing functions.

Under normal conditions, both cementum and bone are covered with other tissues. During passive eruption the gingiva recedes and a small part of the cementum surface may be uncovered. Since cementum is thin near the cervix, and since this tissue is much softer (it contains less mineral) than enamel, the cementum may soon be worn away (toothbrushing) and dentin may become exposed. The uncovered cementum is also extremely susceptible to caries and exceptionally good oral hygiene should be recommended in such cases.

Both cementum and alveolar bone are *calcified connective tissues*. Each has the 3 components commonly found in connective tissues (Table 12–1).

Table 12–1. Components of Cementum and Alveolar Bone

	Cementum	*Alveolar Bone*
1. *Cells*	Cementoblasts	Osteoblasts
	Cementocytes	Osteocytes
	(Cementoclasts)	Osteoclasts
2. *Fibrous matrix*	Collagen fibers	Collagen fibers
3. *Ground substance*	Long carbohydrate chains, attached to protein "backbones"; similar to the ground substance in bone	Long carbohydrate chains, attached to protein "backbones"

In both tissues the fibrous matrix is the dominant component. Both tissues are calcified, which means that hydroxyapatite is present in their fibrous matrix and ground substance. Of the 3 calcified tissues of the tooth, cementum is most comparable with bone, both in appearance and in composition.

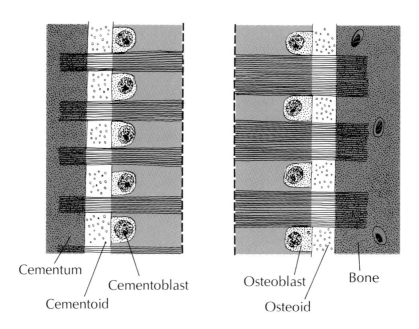

Cementum

Cementoblast

Cementoid

Osteoblast

Bone

Osteoid

Fig. 12–1. Diagram showing the cementum and alveolar bone on either side of a periodontal ligament. Collagen fibers of the periodontal ligament insert into cementum with one end and into bone with the other. More and thinner fiber bundles insert into the cementum than into the alveolar bone. Cementoblasts and osteoblasts line those areas of the cementum and bone surfaces which are located between the inserting fiber bundles. The most recently formed bone and cementum (respectively osteoid and cementoid) layers are noncalcified.

FIBROUS MATRIX

An interesting feature in cementum and alveolar bone is that collagen fibers of the periodontal ligament attach *into* these tissues. During root development, the fibers of the periodontal ligament are synthesized at the same time as the first cementum and alveolar bone are deposited. Gradually, these hard tissues are deposited *around* the ends of the periodontal ligament fibers, embedding them and fixing them in place.

Thus, there are 2 *groups* of *collagen fibers* in cementum and in alveolar bone (Figs. 12–1 and 12–2):

1. Collagen fibers of the *periodontal ligament.* These fibers run into cementum and alveolar bone at an angle that is nearly 90 degrees. These fibers are coarse (somewhat coarser on the alveolar bone side than on the cementum side), and they do not become

Fig. 12–2. The cores of the thicker collagen fibers, which insert into cementum and alveolar bone, remain uncalcified. As a result, they stain less darkly than the surrounding, calcified tissues and remain visible as light "streaks" (Sharpey's fibers) in bone (B) and cementum (C). Original magnification × 40.

completely calcified during the calcification of the surrounding hard tissue. Since the cores of these fibers remain uncalcified, they remain visible, as separate structures, inside the calcified bone or cementum. Any collagen fibers inserting in a calcified tissue anywhere in the body and remaining visible inside the tissue are called *Sharpey's fibers*.

2. Collagen fibers of the *cementum or bone* tissue itself. These collagen fibers are produced by either cementoblasts or osteoblasts as the components of the fibrous matrices of these tissues. They run generally parallel to the dentinocementum junction and to the cementum and bone surfaces, more or less perpendicular to the course of the Sharpey's fibers.

CEMENTUM

Development of Cementum

Cementum can be deposited only after the epithelial root sheath has broken down, allowing cells of the dental sac to move to the surface of the root dentin.

Actually, little cementum is formed until the tooth reaches its functional position in the oral cavity. At that time only two-thirds of the length of the root has been formed. The root surface is covered with a layer of cementoblasts, which are producing cementum. Only a thin layer of mostly uncalcified cementum is actually present at that time.

It has been suggested recently that the epithelial cells of the root sheath, prior to its disintegration, produce some proteins and these are deposited on the surface of the root dentin. Thus, the thin layer of largely uncalcified cementum, which covers the incomplete root at the time of eruption, may consist of cementum matrix produced by the cementoblasts and some of these epithelially produced proteins.

Cementoblasts deposit cementum in a manner similar to the way in which osteoblasts produce bone. They secrete the proteins and the carbohydrate chains of the cementum matrix, while they are moving backward slowly, away from the dentinocementum junction. Once the layer of uncalcified cementum (or *cementoid*) has reached a certain thickness, the earliest formed matrix begins to calcify. From the dentinocementum junction outward, we encounter first calcified cementum, next a strip of cementoid and finally a layer of cementoblasts.

Mature Cementum

The root surface of a fully formed tooth is covered with a cementum layer of uneven thickness and composition.

The cervical half of the root is covered with a thin layer of cementum. At the cervix this cementum may be only 10 μm thick. Although cementoblasts line the surface of the root throughout the functional life of the tooth, little additional deposition of cementum occurs on the cervical half.

In contrast, on the apical half of the root, cementum deposition continues throughout the life of the tooth. Most of this cementum deposition takes place near the apex, where the cementum may reach a thickness of 100 to 150 μm. If the cementum deposition here is excessive, the apical end of the root becomes club-shaped. This is visible in x-ray films, especially of teeth that are no longer in

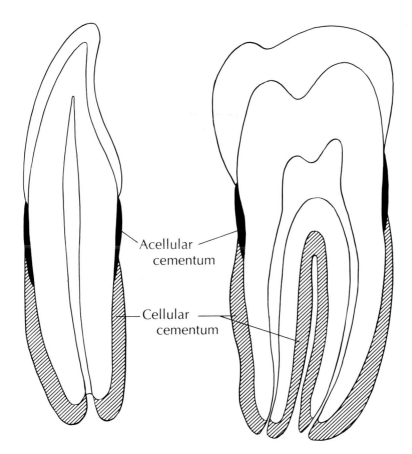

Acellular cementum

Cellular cementum

Fig. 12–3. Diagrams of human teeth, illustrating what parts of the roots are covered with acellular cementum (darkly shaded) or cellular cementum (hatched). The middle of the root may be covered with acellular cementum, overlapped by a layer of cellular cementum. Acellular cementum increases very little in thickness with age. Continuous, slow appositional growth takes place on the cellular cementum surfaces.

functional occlusal contact, because their antagonist (tooth in the opposite jaw) has been lost.

These club-shaped root tips do not give the patients any problems unless extraction of the teeth becomes necessary. In such cases the bony socket may have to be fractured before the tooth can be removed.

The cementum covering the cervical half to two-thirds of the root differs from the cementum covering the apical third of the root, in that the former does not contain any embedded cementocytes (comparable to osteocytes), while the latter does.

The cervical cementum is therefore called *acellular* (or primary, because it forms first in time). The more apically located cementum is called *cellular* (or secondary, because it forms at a later time than primary cementum). All cellular cementum is formed after the tooth has reached functional occlusion. It is not clear which factor(s) may be responsible for the switch from acellular cementum production to cellular cementum production (Fig. 12–3).

During the functional life of a tooth, the width of the *acellular* cementum does *not* increase dramatically. Cementoblasts continue to line this cementum. They are located *between* the inserting fibers of the periodontal ligament. These cells seem to have a role in the maintenance of the existing tissue and only a minor role in new tissue production.

Cellular cementum frequently overlaps acellular cementum on the middle third of the root surface (Fig. 12–4). It contains *cementocytes,* enclosed within cementocytic *lacunae.* These lacunae resemble osteocytic lacunae, with this exception: the cementocytic canaliculi have a preferential orientation toward the periodontal ligament. The periodontal ligament is the only source of nutrition for the cementocytes, which receive this nutrition via their canaliculi. The only exception to this is formed by the cementocytes near the apical foramen. Those cells receive nutrition from the pulpal blood vessels as well (Fig. 12–5).

The *cementoblasts,* which line the cellular cementum, interspersed between the inserting periodontal ligament fibers, have a secretory role. New cementum is deposited throughout life. As is the case with bone deposition, cementum deposition takes place at intervals. When the layer of cementoblasts pauses, a highly calcified layer of cementum is produced. This is an *arrest line.* As in bone, the arrest lines in cementum are smooth (Fig. 12–6).

Reversal lines may be present in cementum, although they are far less abundant than in bone. Cementum undergoes mainly apposition and it does *not* undergo any significant remodeling. However, cementum is not resistant against resorption and an occasional reversal line may be found in nearly all teeth. This means that, at some time during the tooth's presence in the jaw, the conditions were right for cementum resorption, for example, extreme or-acellular

Fig. 12–4. Histologic section, halfway down the length of a dental root. Darkly staining, acellular cementum covers the root dentin (D) and is, in turn, covered by a thick layer of cellular cementum. The dark lines in both types of cementum are arrest lines, comparable to arrest lines in bone. Several cementocytic lacunae, with enclosed cementocytes, are visible in the cellular cementum (arrow). Original magnification × 50.

thodontic movement of teeth, trauma, or dental roots that came too close together (Fig. 12–7).

In such circumstances some resorption (by "cementoclasts," similar in appearance and function to osteoclasts) may occur. When resorption ceases, a highly calcified line forms in the cementum. This line is not smooth, but scalloped, reflecting the final outlines of the resorption cavities. When new cementum is again deposited on this surface, a scalloped reversal line remains, providing us with evidence that resorption did occur.

Since cementum does not undergo any consistent remodeling, this tissue generally becomes thicker with time. This causes some problems for the cementocytes, which are located in the deepest

Fig. 12–5. A comparison between the appearance of osteocytic lacunae in a ground section of lamellar bone (with some parallel lamellae and some osteons), shown in A, and cementocytic lacunae in a ground section of cellular cementum, shown in B. The comparison shows that, at the same magnification, the osteocytic lacunae are grouped much closer together than the cementocytic lacunae. The osteocytic lacunae seem to be arranged more orderly. The small canaliculi, which house the osteocytic cell processes, are oriented in all directions. The cementocytic lacunae, which house the cementocytic cell processes, are oriented preferentially toward the periodontal ligament. Original magnification A and B × 125.

Fig. 12–6.   Darkly staining, smooth arrest lines in cellular cementum (C). This cementum is deposited slowly, throughout life, with long rest intervals. Cementoblasts line the surface of the cementum. Original magnification × 50.

layers of cementum, near the dentinocementum junction. Most osteocytes are no further than 200 μm removed from the nearest blood vessels. In addition, the osteocytic lacunae are extensively interconnected, via their canaliculi, with each other and with the vascular spaces in and around the bone.

The cementocytes tend to be further apart from each other, and their canaliculi do not interconnect quite as richly as the osteocytic canaliculi. All this causes the deepest cementocytes to be slowly deprived of their nourishments and respiratory gases, and these cells perish. It is, therefore, quite normal to find the lacunae near the dentinocementum junction empty.

Fig. 12–7. Scalloped reversal line (arrow), interrupting the regular pattern of arrest lines in cellular cementum. The reversal line represents the final outlines of earlier resorption cavities, which have subsequently been filled (still partially) with repair tissue (cellular cementum). While resorption of cementum is not common in functional teeth, some resorption does occur and most teeth have one or more reversal lines in the cementum. Original magnification × 50.

Cementicles

Abnormal, calcified bodies are occasionally found in the periodontal ligament at some distance from the root surface. These structures are called *cementicles*. It is not completely clear why they form. Generally cementicles seem to form first on cellular debris, such as the epithelial root sheath remnants (cell rests of Malassez). In their appearance, cementicles resemble most the regularly growing false denticles in the dental pulp.

The cementicles may be completely free inside the periodontal ligament. In that case they are called *free cementicles*. Continued cementum deposition on the root surface, as well as on the cementicle's surface, combined with a possible motion of the tooth toward the cementicle, may cause the cementicle to become *attached* to and eventually *embedded* in the cementum layer on the root.

ALVEOLAR BONE

We have already noted that the alveolar bone, which forms the sockets in which the roots of the teeth are suspended, is part of the bone of the jaws. There is no sharp line of division, and we can only designate bone *arbitrarily* as *alveolar bone* versus *basal bone* of the jaw.

Our arbitrary decision is in fact based on clinical experience, especially the cases in which a human being loses all teeth or in which an individual never forms teeth. In the first case we speak of an *edentulous* patient, a candidate for full dentures. In the second case we speak of a totally *anodontic* patient, also a candidate for full dentures.

Following tooth extractions, all alveolar bone gradually is lost in an edentulous patient. This loss is the result of bone resorption, which continues until only the basal bone remains. In the anodontic patient the alveolar bone is never formed.

From these examples it should be clear that alveolar bone depends for its existence entirely on the presence of dental roots (Fig. 12–8). In practice, it also means that full dentures should be checked regularly because they will become looser with the years as more and more alveolar bone (upon which the denture rests) is resorbed.

Gross Appearance of Alveolar Bone

When alveolar bone is inspected with the unaided eye on dental x-ray films (see Chap. 5) or in sectioned bone specimens, the following observations can be made (Fig. 12–9).

1. The cortex of the basal bone of the mandible or maxilla continues as the *cortical plate* of the alveolar bone. We distinguish an *outer cortical plate,* the cortical plate facing the lips and cheeks, and an *inner cortical plate,* the cortical plate facing the tongue or palate. These cortical plates consist of compact, lamellar bone.

2. The actual bone socket around the root is another layer of relatively compact bone. It is called the *cribriform plate.* This gross anatomical term indicates that there are numerous small openings in this bone plate, allowing blood vessels and nerves in the bone and in the periodontal ligament to communicate freely. The cribriform plate is also sometimes called the *lamina dura.* This is an x-ray term, which indicates that this part of the alveolar bone usually shows up as a light line on x-ray films. This, in turn, can lead to the *incorrect* impression that this plate is more calcified than the surrounding bone, making it "harder." Lamina dura literally means hard plate. In fact, the particu-

Fig. 12–8.   Contact x-rays of a lower jaw, with most teeth present, A, and of a lower jaw without teeth, B. The jaws were placed with one surface, indicated with an arrow, flat against the x-ray film. Comparison of the two images reveals how much of the bone is basal bone. In A both basal and alveolar bone are present, while in B no alveolar bone is left. The existence of alveolar bone is related entirely to the presence of teeth.

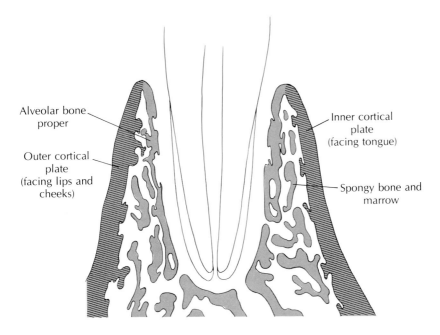

Alveolar bone proper

Outer cortical plate (facing lips and cheeks)

Inner cortical plate (facing tongue)

Spongy bone and marrow

Fig. 12–9. Diagram of a dental root in its alveolar bone socket. The intervening periodontal ligament is not shown. The alveolar bone may be subdivided into a thin plate of alveolar bone proper, which forms the inside wall of the socket, thick, compact plates of cortical bone, on the surfaces of the jaw, and intervening spongy bone. The spaces between the bone trabeculae of the spongy bone are filled with marrow. In young individuals this bone marrow serves as a reservoir for blood cell development (one of many). In older individuals the marrow consists largely of fat.

lar x-ray appearance of the lamina dura is caused by the geometry of this bone plate, rather than by its degree of calcification. Finally, a third name for this bone is *alveolar bone proper,* which simply indicates that this bone constitutes the actual bone socket.

3. Between the cortical plates and the cribriform plate, *spongy bone* may be present. Spongy bone consists of a sparse number of bone trabeculae running inside bone marrow. This bone marrow is originally involved in blood cell production (red marrow, in young individuals), but with age it turns into a predominantly fatty marrow (yellow, rather than red).

Of these gross components, the *essential* one is the alveolar bone proper or *cribriform plate.* The outer cortical plates and the spongy bone may or may not be present. Their role is confined to the support and the streamlining of the cribriform plate (Fig. 12–10, *A*). If a tooth leans toward lips or cheeks, the spongy bone on that side of the tooth is absent and the outer cortical plate is of minimal thickness and fused to the cribriform plate.

Fig. 12–10. A, Alveolar bone, surrounding a premolar. The tooth has been removed to show the anatomy of the socket more clearly. Only a thin plate of alveolar bone proper surrounds the roots, at the side marked with an arrow (facing the cheeks). On the opposite side of the tooth, all 3 components of alveolar bone (alveolar bone proper, spongy bone and a thick, inner cortical plate) are present. The interradicular septum, between the sockets housing the individual roots, is composed of 2 plates of alveolar bone proper (cribriform plates) and an intervening layer of spongy bone. Original magnification × 1. B, X-ray of a ground section through 2 teeth in their alveolar bone sockets. Between the 2 sockets an interdental septum is visible. The septum is composed of 2 cribriform plates (arrows) and an intervening layer of spongy bone. An interdental septum is comparable in structure to an interradicular septum.

The alveolar bone proper, or cribriform plate, houses the single roots and the multiple roots of the various teeth. It forms sockets or *alveoli* around each of these roots. Between the socket of one tooth and the socket(s) of its neighbor, the alveolar bone forms an *interdental septum*. This septum consists of the cribriform plates of both teeth, between which some spongy bone may or may not be present (Fig. 12–10, B).

Similarly, the sockets of two roots of a multi-rooted tooth are separated from each other by an *interradicular septum* (radix means root). This septum consists of the cribriform plates of both roots and, possibly, some spongy bone (Fig. 12–10, A).

Development of Alveolar Bone

Alveolar bone is formed during the development, and especially during the eruption, of the teeth. During the period of dentin and enamel formation, the tooth germs are located in a wide bony groove. This is originally a *common* bony groove for all primary and secondary teeth. Only in late fetal life are small bone septa formed between the different primary teeth. A bony separation between a primary tooth and its secondary successor is formed much later, during the eruption of the primary tooth.

Also during this eruption, most alveolar bone of the primary tooth is formed by deposition of new bone at the rim of the bony groove. This bone grows in *occlusal* direction, along with the erupting tooth, but when the tooth is in functional occlusion, the cervical rim, or rather the *alveolar crest,* of the bone socket remains located slightly more apically than the cervix of the tooth.

The formation of the bony socket around the root of the primary tooth divides the common space in which both primary and secondary teeth were housed before. The secondary successor now lies in a bony *crypt,* which has a small occlusal opening, containing the remnants of the successional dental lamina. One wall of this bony crypt serves also as part of the bony socket of the primary tooth.

With the eruption of the secondary tooth, this common wall is broken down first, and subsequently the secondary tooth erupts through the bony socket of its predecessor. The socket is remodeled extensively to accommodate the (often larger) dimensions of the secondary tooth (Fig. 12–11).

Mature Bone Socket

The cribriform plate of the bone socket (or alveolar bone proper) follows rather precisely the outline of the root surface, which it surrounds. A narrow space, with a thickness of a fraction of a millimeter, is left between the bone and the root. This space is occupied by the periodontal ligament.

The alveolar bone, which started out during development as immature, woven bone, is rapidly remodeled into *lamellar bone* during function. The outer and inner cortical plates are *compact, lamellar* bone, with occasionally a few osteons. Between cribriform plate and cortical plates, *spongy lamellar* bone is present.

The trabeculae of the spongy bone are oriented in 2 principal directions, parallel with and perpendicular to the net direction of the functional loading patterns of this bone. The trabeculae consist of parallel lamellae of bone, without osteons.

A

B

Fig. 12–11. A, The lower jaw of a human fetus, stained with a dye and photographed in transmitted light. No alveolar bone is present as yet in this structure, composed largely of spongy, woven bone. The bony crypts around each of the primary teeth (with their secondary successors) are visible as lighter areas. This is because there is less bone in those areas and the transmitted light passes more easily through them. Original magnification × 5. B, Contact x-ray (original magnification × 1) of the molar region of an adult jaw. The secondary dentition has erupted completely. A second premolar and three molars are visible. The alveolar bone, which surrounds those teeth, has developed largely by bone apposition, in an occlusal direction, on the rims of the original bony crypts, A. In addition, substantial growth has enlarged this part of the jaw to allow enough space for the individual teeth.

272

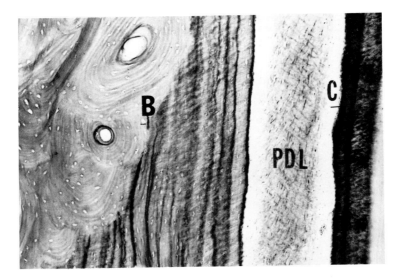

Fig. 12–12. Histologic section through the cribriform plate (alveolar bone proper), which surrounds a tooth. The periodontal ligament (PDL) and the darkly staining cementum (C) on the root surface are to the right of the photograph. The 2 layers of the cribriform plate are seen clearly: the lightly staining compact lamellar bone, with a few osteons, is seen to the left, and the darkly staining bundle bone (B) with several arrest lines. The bundle bone was named for the large number of Sharpey's fibers (light streaks, running obliquely, nearly horizontally) inside the bone matrix. Original magnification × 40.

The cribriform plate itself consists of 2 layers of bone: (1) compact, lamellar bone, with an occasional osteon, and (2) a layer of so-called *bundle bone,* which faces the periodontal ligament. This bone layer is of variable thickness, but always thick enough to anchor the fibers of the periodontal ligament, which insert into this bone layer. The inserting fibers remain visible as *Sharpey's fibers* inside the bone, and they dominate its appearance so much that they are responsible for the name bundle bone (Fig. 12–12).

Remodeling of the Bony Socket

In addition to a small amount of functional, active eruption, the fully erupted teeth may undergo some movements in a horizontal direction. The most common movement is called *mesial drift.* This is a slight movement of all teeth toward the front of the oral cavity. This slight movement occurs at a slow rate, since it depends mostly on wear at the contact points between adjacent teeth. Nevertheless, this movement is frequently substantial enough to make a difference in the appearance of the walls of the bony socket.

Fig. 12–13. Cross section through the roots of 2 adjacent primate teeth with an intervening interdental septum. The section through the interdental septum is made close to the alveolar crest, where the septum is very thin. Consequently, the 2 cribriform plates are very thin (consisting only of bundle bone), and they are fused together, without intervening spongy bone layer. The teeth have been moved orthodontically in the direction of the arrow. As a result, many resorption cavities are present on the left side of the septum, which is in the path of the moving tooth, while massive new bone deposition (2 arrest lines are visible) has taken place on the opposite side of the septum. Original magnification × 40.

If a tooth moves in a certain direction, part of the bone (in the path of the movement) has to be removed to make room for the advancing tooth. In that part of the bony socket you may see osteoclasts inside resorption lacunae (Fig. 12–13). The bone to be broken down first is the bundle bone. The breakdown may result in the detachment of the periodontal fibers, which insert in the bone. However, since the bone resorption is localized, the tooth usually does not become loose.

Occasionally the resorption may extend into the lamellar bone. When enough resorption has taken place, new bone fills in some of the resorption cavities. This new bone re-anchors the fibers of the periodontal ligament, and this bone becomes the new bundle bone.

The side of the bony socket, from which the tooth moves away, does not undergo bone resorption, but rather bone deposition to fill in the distance over which the tooth has moved. In this way the width of the space between the bony socket and the root is kept about the same.

The new bone is deposited around the fibers of the periodontal ligament, and thus it too is of the bundle bone variety. This increases the width of the bundle bone layer at the deposition side. However, continuous bone *remodeling* rapidly removes some of the deeper layers of the bundle bone (the *older* bundle bone) and replaces it with lamellar bone and osteons.

The same remodeling patterns in the bone socket allow the teeth to be moved *orthodontically.* If done properly, orthodontic treat-

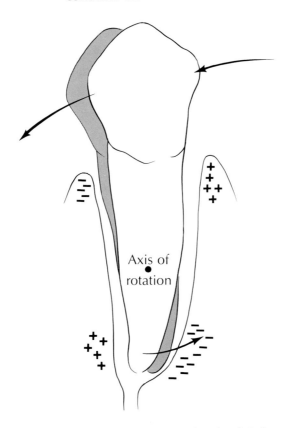

Axis of
● rotation

Fig. 12–14. Orthodontic forces are generally applied to the clinical crown of a tooth, resulting in a tipping movement, with the axis of rotation about midway down the length of the dental root. The alveolar bone reacts to this movement by resorption (−) and deposition (+) in the indicated areas.

ment always is accompanied by bone remodeling, which enables the alveolar bone to accommodate to the new conditions. Most orthodontic movements are tipping movements, leading to corresponding bone remodeling patterns (Fig. 12–14), because orthodontic forces generally can only be applied to the clinical crown of the tooth. The tooth responds by tipping around an axis of rotation located midway down the length of the root.

In addition to bone remodeling to accommodate tooth movements, normal bone remodeling takes place throughout life. The orientation of the bone trabeculae in the spongy bone reflects the loading patterns of the jaw. If the loading conditions are altered, the bone trabeculae are remodeled to adjust to the new conditions. Finally, throughout the body bone remodeling takes place to adjust constantly the circulating levels of calcium and phosphate ions,

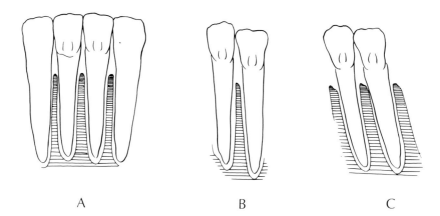

A　　　　　　　　　　B　　　　　　　　　　C

Fig. 12–15.　Under most normal conditions, the tops of the interdental septa, the alveolar crests, are rounded or pointed evenly, A. If 2 adjacent teeth have erupted to unequal vertical positions, B, or if several teeth are slanted, C, the alveolar crests may be slanted. A slanted alveolar crest may indicate the presence of periodontal disease around the tooth at the deep end of the slant. However, when a slanted alveolar crest is noted on an x-ray film, the examples shown in this figure should be remembered and checked.

which are the building blocks of hydroxyapatite, but are also necessary ions for many vital functions.

Shape of the Alveolar Crest

The radiographic image of the top of the interdental septum is used frequently as an indicator of periodontal health or disease. However, some factors may influence the shape of this structure, even in the absence of a pathologic condition.

On dental x-ray films the top of the interdental septum, or the alveolar crest, is normally rounded or pointed evenly. This is the case when the cervices of the 2 adjacent teeth are at the same vertical level.

If one tooth is on a considerably lower level and less erupted, or if both teeth are strongly slanted, the alveolar crest reflects this by being slanted as well. Since slanting is also frequently an indication of periodontal disease, affecting the tooth adjacent to the lowest point of the slanted surface, careful note should be taken of the relationship between the 2 teeth and of their orientation before you decide whether this is a pathologic condition (Fig. 12–15).

SELECTED READING LIST

Furseth, R.: The fine structure of acellular cementum in young human premolars. Scand. J. Dent. Res., *82*:437, 1974.

Giansanti, J.S.: The pattern and width of the collagen bundles in bone and cementum. Oral Surg. Oral Med. Oral Path., 30:508, 1970.

Jones, S.J., and Boyde, A.: A study of human root cementum surfaces as prepared for and examined by electron microscope. Z. Zellforsch., 130:318, 1972.

Melcher, A.H., and Bowen, W.H.: Biology of the Periodontium. New York, Academic Press, 1969.

Owens, P.D.A.: A light microscopic study of the development of the roots of premolar teeth in dogs. Arch. Oral Biol., 19:525, 1974.

Ritchey, B., and Orban, B.: Crests of the interdental alveolar septa. Dent. Radiogr. Photogr., 27:37, 1954.

Ten Cate, A.R.: Formation of supporting bone in association with periodontal ligament organization in the mouse. Arch. Oral Biol., 20:137, 1975.

Updegrave, W.J.: Normal radiographic anatomy. Dent. Radiogr. Photogr., 31:57, 1958.

Chapter 13

PERIODONTAL LIGAMENT

Caries and periodontal disease are the 2 diseases most frequently encountered in dental practice. With the introduction of fluorides and sealants, caries is preventable to a large degree, if not totally. Teeth that are protected against caries now may fall victim to periodontal disease in the future. An understanding of the anatomy and physiology of the periodontal ligament and the dentogingival junction are particularly important in dental practice. We will discuss the periodontal ligament in this chapter and the dentogingival junction in Chapter 14.

The periodontal ligament is a tendon-like structure that ties the tooth to the alveolar bone, to the neighboring teeth and to the gingiva. As we noted in Chapter 12, the 3 tissues responsible for attaching the teeth to the jaw bone (cementum, alveolar bone and periodontal ligament) may be compared with a suspension bridge. If the bone and cementum function as the "towers," the periodontal ligament functions as the cables of the bridge. Neither the towers nor the cables may be removed if the bridge is to remain intact.

As already noted, with the loss of either cementum or alveolar bone the attachment of the tooth fails. Similarly, if the fibers of the periodontal ligament are broken down, for instance by bacterially produced enzymes in periodontal disease, the tooth is lost. A healthy periodontal ligament is yet another key to the survival of the tooth.

The *width* of the periodontal ligament varies somewhat with age, with the functional loading of the tooth, and with its specific location (near the apex or near the cervix of the tooth).

AGE. In younger teenagers, the average width of the periodontal ligament is 0.21 mm. In older people (around 60 years of age) the average width is reduced to 0.15 mm.

LOCATION. In all age groups the periodontal ligament is wider near the cervix and near the apex of the tooth and narrower near the middle of the root. Tipping movements occur during the function of the tooth. These movements consist of rotations around an axis in the middle of the root. This means that any movements in that part of the root (at the level of the axis of rotation) are minimal, but that the movements are greatest near the apex and near the cervix of the tooth. These differences in degree of movement produce the differences in width of the various parts of a periodontal ligament.

FUNCTION. Similarly, an actively functioning tooth has a slightly wider periodontal ligament than a tooth that cannot function, because its antagonist, the tooth in the opposite jaw, is missing.

In *summary,* the width of the periodontal ligament depends on the amount of *use* a tooth gets. The greater the use of a tooth, the greater its tipping movements. If the tooth is used less, because of the absence of its antagonist, or if it is subjected to less movement, because of the wear of the cusps, the width of the ligament is reduced. In older people there may be a loss of teeth and a loss of cusps, leading to less use and fewer movements of the remaining teeth and to a reduction in the width of the periodontal ligament.

TISSUE COMPONENTS OF THE PERIODONTAL LIGAMENT

The periodontal ligament is a product of the cells of the dental sac. These cells, in turn, are derived from neural crest cells. It is a specialized *connective tissue* resembling, both in function and in certain aspects of its histologic appearance, a tendon. The periodontal ligament consists of the 3 components commonly found in connective tissues: (1) *cells* (fibroblasts and other cell types, normally found in connective tissue proper and necessary for the maintenance and the protection of this tissue), (2) *fibrous matrix* (collagen fibers, arranged in dense bundles; delicate oxytalan fibers), and (3) *ground substance* (long carbohydrate chains, attached to protein "backbones" similar to those found in connective tissue proper).

The periodontal ligament consists of a series of heavy collagen fiber bundles. These are called *principal fiber bundles.* They alternate with areas that contain loose connective tissue, blood vessels and nerves. These are called *interstitial areas* (Fig. 13–1).

CELLS. The cells responsible for the production of the fibrous matrix and ground substance of the periodontal ligament are the *fibroblasts.* These are active cells, continuously engaged in secretory activities. The periodontal ligament has a fast turnover rate, probably even faster than that of the lamina propria of the oral mucosa.

New fibrous matrix and ground substance are produced at about the same rate at which the old fibrous matrix and ground substance are broken down. The cells responsible for this breakdown and subsequent digestion of the waste materials appear to be the same

Fig. 13–1. Periodontal ligament of a primate tooth, sectioned lengthwise. The dense, highly organized, collagenous, principal fiber bundles (P) resemble tendon tissue. They alternate with interstitial areas consisting of loose connective tissue. These areas contain the blood vessels and nerves of the periodontal ligament. The arrow points at a small clump of epithelial cells. This is a remnant of the epithelial root sheath. Original magnification × 40.

fibroblasts that are responsible for their production. Thus, the fibroblasts in the periodontal ligament are actively engaged in both secretory and digestive activities. Many fibroblasts have been observed with phagocytic vacuoles, containing fragments of collagen fibers.

Fibroblasts are found both within the principal fiber bundles and in the interstitial areas. When they are located in the fiber bundles, they have the same, typical "squeezed" appearance as fibroblasts in tendons (Fig. 13–2). In cross sections such fibroblasts are

Fig. 13-2. A, Oblique histologic section through the tip of a dental root and several principal fiber bundles (P) of the periodontal ligament (periapical fibers). In this near-cross section, the principal fiber bundles are demonstrably rounded bundles, while the (lighter) interstitial areas form a network, surrounding the bundles. Nuclei of fibroblasts are visible as dark dots in both fiber bundles and interstitial areas. Original magnification × 40. B, A higher magnification of a cross section through collagen fibers in mature tendon tissue. The collagen fibers, seen in cross section (grey), have shrunk, leaving many artificial open spaces between them. The dark dots, squeezed between the fibers, are nuclei of fibroblasts. Some thin cell processes extend between adjacent collagen fibers (arrow). Original magnification × 160.

star-shaped, with their cell bodies, containing little more than the nucleus and a few organelles, squeezed in a cornered space between 3 or more collagen fibers and their cytoplasmic extensions in the narrower spaces between 2 adjacent fibers.

In the interstitial areas, a more diverse group of cells is found. The interstitial areas contain blood vessels and nerves (pp. 286–289), as well as fibroblasts and occasionally other cells, which are commonly found in connective tissue proper (see Chap. 4).

Cementoblasts, occasional cementoclasts, osteoblasts and osteoclasts are physically located inside the periodontal ligament, although they belong, strictly speaking, to the cementum and alveolar bone. The cementoblasts and osteoblasts line the entire lengths of the cementum and bone surfaces, frequently squeezed between the fibers of the periodontal ligament, which insert in these hard tissues.

Osteoclasts usually originate near the blood vessels in the interstitial areas, and the bone next to these areas is, more often than not, the first to be resorbed.

Finally, in the periodontal ligaments of newly erupted teeth, small clusters and cords of epithelial cells may be found parallel to, but at some distance from, the root surface. These are the *epithelial remnants* (Malassez) of the root sheath. Generally, these groups of cells are inactive though they are alive. Each group or cord is surrounded by its own basal lamina, which separates the epithelial cells from the surrounding connective tissues. No function has been attributed to these cell groups and cell death slowly reduces their numbers. The suggestion has been made that cellular debris of these remnants may stimulate the formation of cementicles, but there is no complete, adequate proof of this.

FIBROUS MATRIX. The dominant components of the periodontal ligament are its collagenous *principal fiber* bundles. These bundles all insert into the cementum, covering the root, and run from there into the lamina propria of the gingiva, the periosteum, covering the outer cortical plate of the alveolar bone, the cementum of a neighboring tooth, and, most importantly, directly into the alveolar bone proper.

The fibers inserting into the alveolar bone are somewhat coarser than the ones inserting into the cementum. The 2 groups of fibers meet midway, across the width of the periodontal ligament, where they are interconnected with each other.

The principal fiber bundles may be arranged in the following distinct groups (Figs. 13–3 and 13–4):

1. *Gingival Fibers.* These fibers run from the most cervical cementum into the gingiva (lamina propria). Some may actually run *over* the alveolar crest into the lamina propria of the attached gingiva and into the periosteum of the cortical plates.

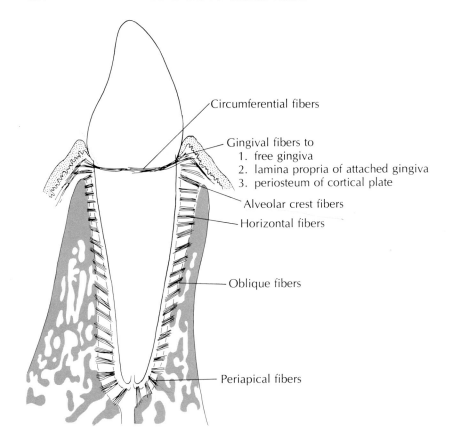

Fig. 13–3. *Diagram of a human tooth (lingual side to the left, side facing lips and cheeks to the right). The various principal fiber groups are indicated. Circumferential fibers are shown in three dimensions. They insert in the most cervical cementum, run partially around the dental root, and insert either in the gingival lamina propria or in the bone of the alveolar crest. All other fiber groups are shown in only 2 dimensions (as if they are sectioned). About two-thirds of the length of the root is suspended by oblique fibers.*

2. *Circumferential Fibers.* These fibers originate in the most cervical cementum and run horizontally around and parallel to part of the root. Some fibers insert into the lamina propria of the gingiva. Others insert into the alveolar crest.

3. *Transseptal Fibers.* These fibers run from the cementum of one tooth, *over* the top of the interdental septum, into the cementum of the next tooth.

4. *Alveolar Crest Fibers.* These fibers run from the cementum of the tooth, in an apically slanted direction, to the alveolar crest, where they insert.

5. *Horizontal Fibers.* These fibers run, in a horizontal direction,

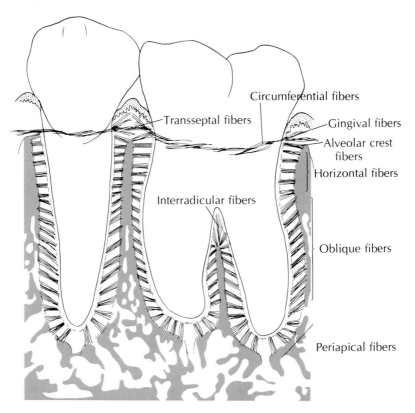

Circumferential fibers

Transseptal fibers

Gingival fibers

Alveolar crest fibers

Horizontal fibers

Interradicular fibers

Oblique fibers

Periapical fibers

Fig. 13–4. Diagram of 2 adjacent human teeth, separated by an interdental septum. Compared with Fig. 13–3, two additional fiber groups are visible in this view. Transseptal fibers run from one tooth to the next over the interdental septum. Interradicular fibers run from the tip of the interradicular septum in a radiating pattern into the furcation area between the roots.

from the cementum covering the cervical third of the root toward the alveolar bone, where they insert.

6. *Oblique Fibers.* These fibers run from the cementum covering the apical two-thirds of the root, in an occlusally slanted direction, toward the bone, into which they insert.

7. *Periapical Fibers.* These fibers run, in a radiating fashion, from the cementum of the apex toward the alveolar bone, where they insert.

8. *Interradicular Fibers* (in *multirooted* teeth *only*). These fibers run from the cementum in the furcation area (the concave area where the bases of the roots meet), converging toward the top of the interradicular septum of the alveolar bone.

It is clear from the foregoing list that the periodontal fibers, which insert into the cementum all along the root of the tooth, tie the tooth to *all* surrounding structures. The orientations of the fiber bundles are varied, giving the tooth optimal resistance to all types of loading.

In addition to resisting all types of loading, the principal fiber bundles transform the compressive loadings produced on the tooth during chewing into evenly distributed tension on the alveolar bone. Since bone is particularly resistant to *tensile* loadings (see Chap. 5), this is an effective mechanical arrangement.

For example, the oblique fibers resist occlusal loadings; the circumferential fibers resist rotational movements of the tooth; the alveolar crest fibers and the periapical fibers resist pull of the tooth from the socket.

The transseptal fibers connect all teeth and are responsible for the maintenance of the uninterrupted dental arch. Once a single tooth has been lost, the integrity of the dental arch is disturbed, and the remaining segments behave as independent units.

A delicate network of *oxytalan* fibers is also present within the periodontal ligament. Some of these fibers run parallel to the root surface; others insert into the cementum. While the function of these fibers is not clear, it has been postulated that they serve as a supporting network for the blood vessels in the periodontal ligament.

BLOOD VESSELS

A tooth, its periodontal ligament, and its alveolar bone have a common blood supply. Each tooth and its periodontium are supplied by one small artery, which runs as a branch from the main arterial supply in the jaw toward the apical foramen of the tooth (Fig. 13–5). Before it enters this foramen, the artery gives off a group of small arteriolar branches to supply the alveolar bone, and a second group of branches to supply the periodontal ligament all around the tooth. The remaining artery branches once more into a few arterioles, which finally enter the pulp through the apical foramen (Fig. 13–6).

The blood vessels supplying the pulp tissue have no further connection with the other blood vessels outside the tooth. This means that when the arterioles to the dental pulp are cut accidentally, the pulp no longer receives any vascular supply and perishes.

The arterioles supplying the alveolar bone, on the other hand, have many connections with each other, and if one blood vessel is cut, others take over its functions. The arterioles supplying the periodontal ligament are also richly interconnected with each other. All these vessels run inside the netlike structure of interstitial areas. The blood vessels lie closer to the surface of the alveolar bone than to the cementum surface.

The vascular networks of periodontal ligament and alveolar bone form many connections with each other. The connecting blood

*Fig. 13–5. Section through the bony canal (arrows), which contains the blood vessels and nerves, supplying a single tooth and its surrounding tissues. Original magnification ×
10.*

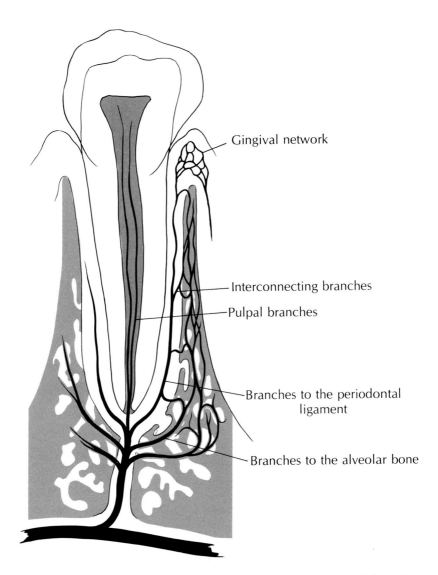

Gingival network

Interconnecting branches

Pulpal branches

Branches to the periodontal
ligament

Branches to the alveolar bone

*Fig. 13–6.   Diagram showing schematically the pattern of the vascular (arterial) supply to
a human tooth and surrounding tissues. A single artery branches off the main arterial
supply of the jaw (bottom). From this artery, several branches supply the alveolar bone all
around the socket. In addition, several branches supply the periodontal ligament all
around the root. Finally, the remaining artery subdivides into a few pulpal branches, which
enter the tooth through the apical foramen. Notice the numerous interconnecting
branches between blood vessels of the periodontal ligament and the alveolar bone. A
particularly extensive vascular network is present in the gingiva. It is formed by
interconnecting branches of the gingival blood vessels, periodontal blood vessels and
alveolar bone blood vessels.*

vessels cross the cribriform plate via the several small openings, which give the cribriform plate its name.

Venous drainage pathways roughly parallel the arterial supply pathways. A particularly extensive venous network is present in the periodontal ligament surrounding the apex of the tooth.

NERVES

The periodontal ligament contains 2 types of nerves: (1) autonomic, sympathetic nerve fibers, which run parallel with the blood vessels and regulate the blood flow in the microvascular beds; and (2) afferent, sensory nerves, which are mostly myelinated branches of the second and third divisions of the fifth cranial nerve (trigeminal nerve). The periodontal ligament is extremely richly supplied with these afferent fibers. Two types of nerve endings are found: (1) *free*, uncovered nerve endings, and (2) *encapsulated* nerve endings.

The free nerve endings appear to be responsible for pain sensation, while the encapsulated endings register pressure changes. The encapsulated endings are far less complicated structures than the ones found in the skin and in the oral mucosa. However, their large numbers are responsible for the delicate perceptive abilities of the periodontal ligament.

Place a thin piece of paper between your teeth and notice how aware you are of its presence. This should be remembered when a restoration is finished. If the "bite" is too high, the patient certainly is sensitive to this. Follow the indications of the patient to improve the restoration. The patient's perception may be more precise than your own observations, in this case.

DEVELOPMENT OF THE
PERIODONTAL LIGAMENT

During the early stages of tooth development, the enamel organ is surrounded by the neural crest-derived dental sac. Because of its arrangement *around* the *expanding* enamel organ, and because collagen fibers tend to be oriented along lines of tension, the cells of the dental sac, and the first fibers they synthesize, assume an orientation *parallel to the outer surface* of the *enamel organ*. This situation persists until the root begins to develop and the tooth is erupting.

At that time, a few of the fibers of the dental sac, while retaining their orientation parallel to the enamel organ and crown surfaces, insert with one end into the developing, most cervical part of the cementum. Around the developing root, some of the dental sac fibers remain oriented parallel to the root surface. However, the dental sac cells closest to the root surface, as well as those closest to

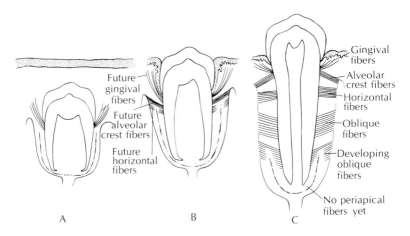

Fig. 13–7. *Stages in the development of the periodontal ligament of a tooth: A, Early during active, prefunctional eruption; B, during emergence of the tooth into the oral cavity; C, upon reaching functional occlusion. A single line, parallel to the surface of the root, and running around the developing apex, reflects the orientation of the dental sac fibers. Those are gradually replaced, in a direction from cervix to apex, by the principal fiber bundles, which are characteristic for a functioning tooth.*

the bone surface, differentiate into fibroblasts and begin to produce collagen fibers. These fibroblasts arrange themselves in rows oriented *perpendicularly* to the surfaces of the root and the bony crypt. The short collagen fibers produced by these cells assume the same orientation, perpendicular to the hard tissue surfaces (Fig. 13–7).

All this takes place first near the cervix, and as the root develops further, the processes of fibroblast differentiation and fiber production gradually move further apically. The more cervically produced fibers, meanwhile, grow longer and soon meet their opposite counterparts, the fibers produced at the bone surface.

When the 2 groups of fibers meet, connections are established between them in a so-called *intermediate plexus,* and a principal fiber bundle is formed. Initially, the fiber bundles have an oblique orientation, similar to the orientation of the later formed oblique fiber group. They run from the developing root in an occlusal direction, toward the bone (Fig. 13–7). With further eruption of the tooth, this orientation is changed by the altered position of the tooth, relative to the bone. This change is most striking for the alveolar crest fibers, which become slanted in an opposite direction, and less striking for the horizontal fibers, which change only from an oblique to a horizontal orientation. The oblique fiber group is established only toward the end of the eruptive period and these keep their oblique orientation. The periapical fibers, of course, are the last to be formed.

SELECTED READING LIST

Freeman, E., and Ten Cate, A.R.: Development of the periodontium: An electron microscopic study. J. Periodontol., 42:387, 1971.

Fullmer, H.M.: Connective tissue components of the periodontium. In *Structural and Chemical Organization of Teeth.* Vol. II. Edited by A.E.W. Miles. New York, Academic Press, 1967.

Grant, D., and Bernick, S.: Formation of the periodontal ligament. J. Periodontol., 43:17, 1972.

Hindle, M.O.: The intermediate plexus of the periodontal membrane. In *The Mechanisms of Tooth Support.* Edited by D.J. Anderson. Bristol, John Wright and Sons, 1967.

Levy, B.M., Dreizen, S., and Bernick, S.: *The Marmoset Periodontium in Health and Disease.* Basel, S. Karger, 1972.

Listgarten, M.A.: Intracellular collagen fibrils in the periodontal ligament of the mouse, rat, hamster, guinea pig and rabbit. J. Periodont. Res., 8:335, 1973.

Melcher, A.H., and Bowen, W.H.: *Biology of the Periodontium.* New York, Academic Press, 1969.

Severson, J.A., Moffett, B.C., Kokich, V., and Selipsky, H.: A histologic study of age changes in the adult human periodontal joint (ligament). J. Periodontol., 49:189, 1978.

Sims, M.R.: Oxytalan-vascular relationships observed in histologic examination of the periodontal ligaments of man and mouse. Arch. Oral Biol., 20:713, 1975.

Sims, M.R.: Oxytalan meshwork associations observed histologically in the periodontium of the mouse mandible. Arch. Oral Biol., 22:605, 1977.

Ten Cate, A.R., and Deporter, D.A.: The role of the fibroblast in collagen turnover in the functioning periodontal ligament of the mouse. Arch. Oral Biol., 19:339, 1974.

Tonna, E.A.: Histological age changes associated with mouse parodontal tissues. J. Gerontol., 28:1, 1973.

Chapter 14

DENTOGINGIVAL JUNCTION

The dentogingival junction is the junction between the gingival epithelium and the tooth surface. The particular nature of this junction makes it a rather vulnerable structure, which is fairly easily disturbed. Once the dentogingival junction *is* disturbed, for instance by the presence of dental plaque or calculus, the underlying connective tissue and the periodontium: bone, cementum and periodontal ligament, are easily invaded by microorganisms, and periodontal disease may result. If not checked, this disease may ultimately lead to the demise of the tooth. The microorganisms and their products destroy the periodontal ligament's fibers and cause resorption of the alveolar bone.

A healthy dentogingival junction is therefore the key to a healthy periodontium, which in turn is an important factor in the life expectancy of a tooth.

In this chapter the *development* of the component parts of the dentogingival junction, the gingiva and the cervical area of the tooth, will be described, as will the *mature morphology* of this junction.

DEVELOPMENT OF THE JUNCTIONAL EPITHELIUM OF THE GINGIVA

1. *PERIOD PRIOR TO THE TOOTH'S EMERGENCE INTO THE ORAL CAVITY.* Following the completion of enamel formation, the remnant of the enamel organ, the reduced enamel epithelium, continues to cover the anatomical crown of the tooth. The ameloblasts are still lying next to their finished product. At this time, the outermost layer of the enamel is not yet completely calcified. No structure intervenes between the ameloblasts and the partially calcified enamel matrix.

2. *PERIOD OF TOOTH EMERGENCE.* During tooth eruption, the reduced enamel epithelium consists of a thin, non-keratinized, stratified squamous epithelium. A basal lamina sepa-

293

rates the outer epithelial cells from the surrounding connective tissue. The epithelial cells produce enzymes, breaking down the connective tissues between them and the oral epithelium. As the tooth approaches the oral epithelium, the basal laminae of reduced enamel epithelium and of oral epithelium fuse first, then centrally disintegrate. This disintegration is followed by a fusion of the epithelia themselves. The epithelial cells, which are located in the center of this fused mass, disintegrate, and this establishes an opening through which the crown of the tooth emerges into the oral cavity (Fig. 14–1, A, B).

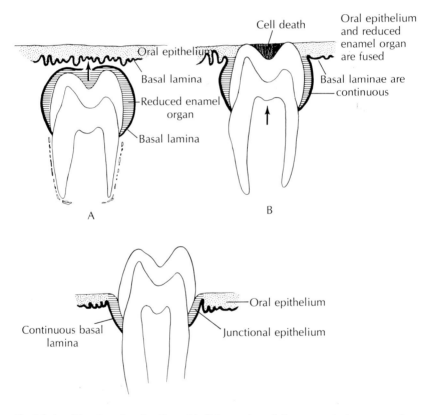

Fig. 14–1. *Diagrams showing the epithelial covering of the anatomical crown surface prior to the tooth's emergence in the oral cavity, A, during the tooth's emergence into the oral cavity, B, and following the tooth's emergence into the oral cavity, C. Prior to emergence the reduced enamel organ (shaded with horizontal lines) approaches the oral epithelium (stippled) and is subsequently fused with it. Cell death occurs in the center of the fused epithelium, B. This results in the development of an opening through which the tooth emerges. The first junctional epithelium of the dentogingival junction is the most cervical part of the reduced enamel organ, C.*

3. *PERIOD FOLLOWING THE TOOTH'S EMERGENCE INTO THE ORAL CAVITY.* As the tooth erupts further, more and more enamel is uncovered. However, when functional occlusion is reached, a small strip of reduced enamel epithelium, *including the ameloblasts,* still covers the most cervical enamel (Fig. 14–1, C).

This epithelium, which is fused with the oral epithelium, constitutes the *first junctional epithelium* of the dentogingival junction. Secondarily, some time after the tooth has reached functional occlusion, the non-ameloblastic cells of the reduced enamel epithelium begin to proliferate, replacing all the older cells of the reduced enamel epithelium, *including* the ameloblasts, which formed the first attachment to the tooth surface. The newly proliferated cells now establish the *definitive junctional epithelium.*

As the enamel surface matures and becomes completely calcified, the junctional epithelial cells produce a *basal lamina* on this surface.

DEVELOPMENT OF THE CERVIX OF THE TOOTH

The cervix of the tooth marks the borderline between anatomical crown and anatomical root. Theoretically, this border should be a fine line where enamel and cementum meet in an edge-to-edge relationship. In practice, this type of *cemento-enamel junction* is present in only 30% of all teeth. In 60% of the teeth, a strip of cementum overlaps a small part of the enamel, whereas in 10% of all teeth, enamel and cementum do not meet, leaving a strip of dentin uncovered (Fig. 14–2).

These various types of cemento-enamel relationships can only be understood when the development of this region is reviewed (see Chap. 9). There are a few distinct differences in the development of anatomical crown and root:

1. The anatomical crown is shaped by a *complex* epithelial enamel organ, consisting of 4 distinct layers. The anatomical root is shaped by the epithelial root sheath, consisting *only* of a continuation of outer and inner enamel epithelium.

2. Following the induction of the odontoblasts, the inner enamel epithelial cells in the enamel organ differentiate *themselves* into enamel-producing cells, the ameloblasts. The cells of the epithelial root sheath do not appear to have any further function after the shaping of the root and the induction of the root odontoblasts.

3. Following all of its activities, the remnant of the enamel organ, the reduced enamel epithelium, must continue to *cover* the enamel surface until the anatomical crown emerges (partially) into the oral cavity. If the reduced enamel epithelium falls apart *before* eruption is completed, the enamel surface, exposed to the surrounding connective tissues, is soon covered by a layer of cementum, produced by

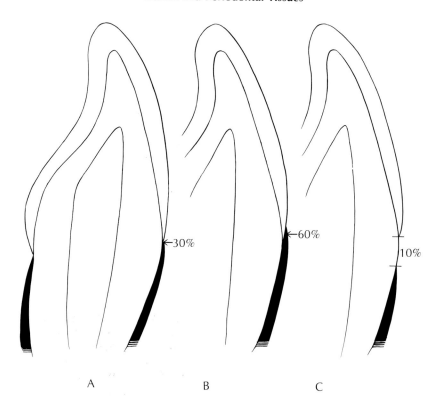

←30%

←60%

10%

A

B

C

Fig. 14–2. Diagram showing 3 possible relationships between enamel (blank) and cementum (black) at the cervix of the tooth. In 30% of all cases an edge-to-edge relationship is present, A. In 60% of all cases the cementum overlaps a small part of the enamel cap, B. In 10% of all cases enamel and cementum do not meet, leaving a strip of uncovered dentin, C.

newly differentiated cementoblasts. Occasionally, when a tooth fails to erupt, this is precisely what happens. The cementum-covered crown of such an *impacted* tooth becomes eventually attached to the surrounding bony crypt walls. In *contrast,* the epithelial root sheath *must* fall apart in order for the cementoblasts to differentiate and move to the root surface, to begin producing cementum.

The last-mentioned point is critical to the development of the cemento-enamel junction. If the anatomical crown retains its epithelial cover while the anatomical root loses its epithelial cover, a perfect edge-to-edge relationship between enamel and cementum is established.

However, in 60% of all cases, the most cervical part of the reduced enamel epithelium breaks down along with the epithelial root sheath. In these cases, cementoblasts cover the exposed strip of cervical enamel with cementum, creating an overlap of cementum over enamel.

Rather less frequently, in about 10% of all cases, the most cervical part of the epithelial root sheath continues to exist intact, together with the reduced enamel epithelium. In such cases cementoblasts are not able to move in, underneath this epithelium, and no cementum is deposited. This leaves a narrow strip of uncovered dentin at the cervix.

Following eruption, the *first* junctional epithelium of the dentogingival junction consists of whatever part of reduced enamel epithelium still covers the tooth surface. In both the knife-edge cemento-enamel junction and the overlap junction (a total of 90%) the first junctional epithelium is in contact with the most cervical, noncementum-covered *enamel* only.

In 10% of all cases, the first junctional epithelium is in contact with the most cervical enamel *plus* the strip of uncovered dentin.

MORPHOLOGY OF THE DENTOGINGIVAL JUNCTION

The fully developed dentogingival junction is formed by an extension of the gingiva, which bends over at the crest of the free gingiva and then faces the surface of the tooth. *All* gingival epithelium, which faces the tooth, we call *dentogingival epithelium*. It consists of nonkeratinized, stratified squamous epithelium. It is subdivided into 2 parts: a *sulcular* part, which is located more occlusally, at the level of the free gingiva (*sulcular epithelium*), and a deeper part (*junctional epithelium*), which closely adheres to the tooth surface.

The sulcular part of the dentogingival epithelium stands away from the enamel surface, forming a shallow sulcus, all around the tooth, with the tooth surface. The 0.5 mm deep sulcus is lined with the sulcular epithelium (nonkeratinized, stratified squamous). The floor of this sulcus is at about the same level as the free gingival groove on the outside (keratinized) surface of the gingiva. Thus, the edge of the sulcus is formed by free gingiva.

When the depth of the sulcus is probed clinically, the probe frequently is pushed down, far beyond the floor of the anatomical sulcus, through the entire junctional epithelium. In doing this, we create our own clinical sulcus by tearing the epithelium itself. This is possible because the epithelial cells, which form an attachment to the enamel surface, remain attached to it (Fig. 14–3). This exercise demonstrates that the attachments between different epithelial cells are broken down more easily than the attachments between epithelial cells and the enamel surface.

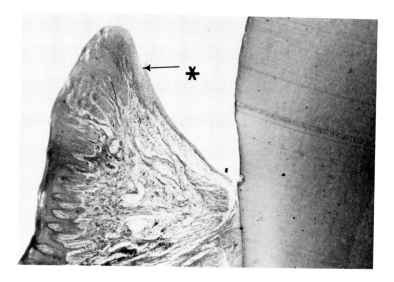

Fig. 14–3. *The dentogingival junction in a decalcified histologic section of a human tooth. No enamel is visible; it was formerly located in the space marked with an asterisk, but was lost during decalcification. The epithelium of the gingiva, which faces the space, is dentogingival epithelium. The floor of the gingival sulcus is indicated* (arrow). *The epithelium above it is sulcular epithelium, while the epithelium below it is junctional epithelium. The interface between junctional epithelium and underlying connective tissue is smooth. Several gingival fiber bundles are visible in this section. Some run into the free gingiva, others run into the lamina propria of the attached gingiva. Original magnification* × 12.5.

The *junctional epithelium* forms hemidesmosomal contacts with the basal lamina, which it has deposited on the enamel surface. The nature of this attachment is therefore similar to the nature of the attachment between an epithelium and the underlying connective tissue (Fig. 14–4).

Since the junctional epithelium faces enamel on one side and connective tissue on the other side, it is sandwiched between 2 basal laminae, which are continuous with each other, around the most cervical edge of the junctional epithelium.

Cell renewal takes place in the basal cells of the epithelium, where it faces the connective tissue, and in the most cervical cells as well. The newly proliferated cells move slowly in an occlusal direction, toward the oral cavity, where the older cells are sloughed off.

Mechanically the dentogingival attachment is strong. The basal lamina adheres to the dental enamel and the junctional epithelial cells adhere to the basal lamina. This adhesion is enhanced by capillary action, which keeps these structures together, rather like 2 glass plates with a thin film of liquid between them.

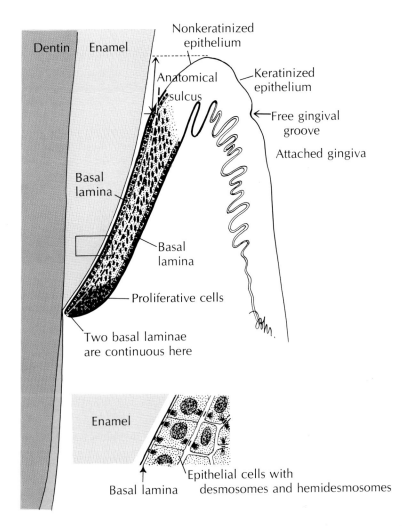

Fig. 14–4. Schematic diagram of the dentogingival epithelium. The nature of the attachment between junctional epithelium and tooth surface is shown in more detail in the insert. A basal lamina adheres to the tooth surface, while the junctional epithelial cells, in turn, form hemidesmosomal attachment plaques on the basal lamina. The free gingival groove and the floor of the anatomical sulcus are at the same vertical level. Careless clinical probing may lead to the establishment of a "clinical sulcus" (which will, under normal conditions, heal rapidly) along the broken line indicated in this diagram.

With age, the junctional epithelium may recede apically and migrate onto the root surface, exposing more of the crown of the tooth. This is the process of *passive eruption.* The dentogingival junction is formed originally by the junctional epithelium and the enamel surface. With age, it may become an attachment between the junctional epithelium and both enamel *and* cementum surfaces. Ultimately, the attachment may become located *entirely* on the cementum surface.

Gingival recession may be sped up by an inflammation of the gingiva. Inflammation is generally brought about by microorganisms in the dental plaque. Clinically, an inflamed gingiva becomes swollen and red. Histologically, *large numbers* of inflammatory cells are present in the gingival connective tissue. (Even in healthy gingivae *some* lymphocytes are usually present underneath the junctional epithelium.)

The inflammation process leads to a breakdown of the dentogingival attachment and a real deepening of the gingival sulcus. Apical downward proliferation of the cervical-most epithelial cells follows, and the entire attachment is displaced apically. Once substantial apical proliferation has taken place, treatment frequently must include periodontal surgery, removing much of the free gingiva to reduce the depth of the gingival sulcus.

INVESTMENTS OF THE TOOTH
SURFACE

The dentogingival attachment is frequently complicated by the presence of a thin *cuticle,* located between the surface of the tooth and the basal lamina, associated with the junctional epithelial cells. The *dental cuticle* has an unknown composition. It is first formed during late eruption, probably by the reduced ameloblasts.

If a newly erupted tooth is placed in a 10% solution of hydrochloric acid, a delicate membrane floats off the surface in approximately 2½ hours. This membrane is called *Nasmyth's membrane,* and it consists of a thin dental cuticle with some cells of the reduced enamel organ adhering to it.

With age, the dental cuticle slowly increases in thickness, and it is best seen, with a light microscope, in a section through the dentogingival junction of an older person, in which it may exceed a thickness of 1.0 μm (Fig. 14–5).

BLOOD VESSELS

The *gingiva* around the neck of a tooth receives an especially rich vascular supply. The gingival vascular network is formed by interconnecting blood vessels from 3 different sources: the periodontal ligament, the alveolar bone and the periosteum of the cortical plates

Fig. 14–5. Dental cuticle (between arrows) located between the root surface (acellular cementum) and the junctional epithelium. There is an abundance of inflammatory cells (dark dots) in the gingival tissues. These cells partially mask the receded junctional epithelium and the fiber bundles underneath it. Original magnification × 50.

(see Fig. 13–6). The periosteum, in turn, is supplied by branches of the blood vessels inside the bone and in the muscles attaching to the bone surface.

Venous drainage pathways roughly parallel the arterial supply pathways. An extensive venous network is present in the gingiva around the neck of the tooth.

This extensive blood vessel supply should be remembered when you deal clinically with this critically important region of the gingiva and the dentogingival junction.

SELECTED READING LIST

Armitage, G.C., and Christie, T.M.: Structural changes in exposed human cementum.
I. Light microscopic observations. J. Period. Res., *8*:343, 1973.

Armitage, G.C., and Christie, T.M.: Structural changes in exposed human cementum. II. Electron microscopic observations. J. Period. Res., 8:356, 1973.

Brady, J.M., and Woody, R.D.: Scanning microscopy of cervical erosion. J.A.D.A., 94:726, 1977.

Kobayashi, K., Rose, G.C., and Mahan, C.J.: Ultrastructure of the dentoepithelial junction. J. Period. Res., 11:313, 1976.

Löe, H.: The structure and physiology of the dentogingival junction. In Structural and Chemical Organization of Teeth. Vol. II. Edited by A.E.W. Miles. New York, Academic Press, 1967.

Newman, H. N.: The pre-eruptive portion of the human enamel integument. J. Dent., 3:110, 1975.

Schroeder, H.E., and Listgarten, M.A.: Fine Structure of the Developing Epithelial Attachment of Human Teeth. Basel, S. Karger, 1971.

Taylor, A.C., and Campbell, M.M.: Reattachment of gingival epithelium to the tooth. J. Periodontol., 43:281, 1972.

Appendix **I**

USE OF THE MICROSCOPE

One of the most important aspects of studying histology is the art of making careful observations with the microscope. Here are a few guidelines for the use of the light microscope (Fig. A–1).

1. Make sure that the lenses in the *eyepiece, objectives* and *condenser* are clean at all times. To prevent scratching of these valuable lenses, use special lens paper for cleaning.

2. Place a glass slide on the microscope *stage* and clamp it into place.

3. Turn on the light source at the base of the microscope.

4. Looking through the eyepiece, inspect the slide. Turn first the *coarse adjustment,* then the *fine adjustment,* until the image is clear (focused).

5. Now, turn the lever of the *iris diaphragm,* until almost all the light is *blocked.*

6. With the diaphragm in this closed position, turn the *condenser adjustment* until you see (through the eyepiece) a sharp edge between the diaphragm's shadow and the central light area. This means that the light beam passing through your glass slide is also *focused* properly.

7. Remove your eyepiece and look directly down into the *body tube* of the microscope. Now, slowly *open the diaphragm,* just until you see, at the base of the tube, a clear light field, from which the edge of the diaphragm's shadow has disappeared. Do *not* open the diaphragm any further, or you will lose some of the light, which should be passing through the specimen on the stage.

8. *Replace the eyepiece* and hold a sheet of white paper over it. The light, which comes through the body tube and out of the eyepiece, will make a sharp light dot on the paper when you hold it about $1/3$ to $1/2$ inch away from the eyepiece.

This *should be the position* of your eye during the use of the microscope.

The microscope is now optimally adjusted for study.

Fig. A–1.   The light path through the various lenses of a monocular microscope (with only one eyepiece) is shown. The light beam may come directly from a light source at the base of the microscope or it may be reflected by a mirror, as is shown here. The various parts of the microscope are clearly indicated on this photograph/diagram. From the base upward : condenser lenses, with condenser adjustment (control knob) and the lever (control) of the iris diaphragm; the stage with the object (illustrated here by an arrow). The object usually is mounted on a glass slide, which in turn is clamped firmly to the stage by stage clips. There are several objectives (lenses), for different magnifications, mounted in a revolving nosepiece. The entire tube of the microscope may be moved up and down by coarse adjustment and fine adjustment (focusing knobs). The approximately correct position of the eye, relative to the lenses in the eyepiece, is demonstrated. (The Wolfe microscope, path of light, kindly supplied by Carolina Biological Supply Company, Burlington, North Carolina.)

Appendix II

HISTOLOGIC TECHNIQUE

The light microscope, in its simplest form, was first developed around 1600 A.D. The instrument has undergone many refinements since.

The Englishman Robert Hooke and the Dutchman Anthony van Leeuwenhoeck were among the earliest microscopists, who with great curiosity looked at a variety of microscopical structures and described them meticulously. This took place in the Seventeenth Century. Their ingenuity and accuracy of description made the scientific world at that time familiar with structures such as the eyes of a fly, chips of plants, wood, cork, sand and the various microorganisms that could be found in drops of fresh water.

It soon became clear that any object studied with the microscope had to be thin, so as to allow the light to pass through it. To illustrate this point, try to make a thin section of a plant leaf. When you study such a handcut section by light microscopy, you will find that only in the thin areas of the section is any structure at all visible.

Also remember your experiment (Chap. 3), in which you studied whole cells from your own oral mucosa. Few details could be seen in those cells. If you could have cut the cells in half, stained them and made them transparent, you would have seen many more details. It has been found that ideally, for light microscopic purposes, we need sections that are thinner than the diameters of individual cells.

In the Nineteenth Century a great many improvements were made in the optics of the light microscope and, simultaneously, improvements were made in the preparation of the specimens. Machines (microtomes) were developed to cut rather thin sections, and the microscopists began to use a number of stains (originally dyes from the cloth dying industries) to highlight and identify various components of cells and tissues. The discipline of *histology* was now established as an independent branch of the morphologic sciences.

On the following pages, you will find a simple description of the basic steps in specimen preparation, as used at present for simple light microscopy.

305

A tissue for microscopic study may be taken from a living individual *(biopsy)* or from an individual who has recently died *(necropsy)*. Soon after death, the process of tissue breakdown begins (as the result of lysosomal enzyme release). It is therefore important to take a necropsy specimen at the earliest possible time, so that the tissues still resemble the living state.

FIXATION

Every histologic specimen needs fixation. Fixation is a process in which the structures of tissues and cells are preserved, as much as possible, in the position they occupy during life. While there are several modes of fixation, depending on subsequent treatments of the tissue or the preference of the histologist, the standard fixative for most routine histologic work is a 10% formaldehyde solution. Fixation time varies from 24 hours to several days, depending on the size of the specimen.

Other frequently used fixation methods include the use of a high percentage of alcohol and, for temporary fixation, the freezer.

EMBEDDING

In order to make sections thin enough, the specimen, which is rather soft, has to be hardened, usually by embedding it in *paraffin*. The process of embedding is designed in such a way that all the water inside and outside the various tissue components is *replaced* with paraffin. Since water and paraffin do not mix, this cannot be done by placing the specimen in melted paraffin immediately after fixation. Intermediate steps are required.

After fixation, the specimen is "run through" an "alcohol series," a series of alcohol solutions of increasing strength: 50%, 70%, 96% and 100%. The total length of time that a specimen spends in the alcohol series varies from one-half to 2 days. Alcohol replaces water in the tissues, and by the time the tissues come out of the 100% alcohol, no water remains in them. In the next steps the alcohol is gradually replaced with xylene, which in turn is replaced with warm, melted paraffin.

When all alcohols and xylenes are replaced with paraffin, the paraffin is cooled and allowed to harden in a block around the specimen. This paraffin block is mounted in a holder and placed in a microtome.

SECTIONING

The hardness of the paraffin is well suited to make sections 5 to 10 μm thick. During the sectioning process the sections may become slightly folded and they are stretched in a warm water bath, following which a section is "glued" to a glass slide. If nothing else is done to this section, it will be hard to see any detail under the microscope, owing to the presence of the paraffin and the absence of color of the tissue.

Therefore, the paraffin must be removed in xylene, followed by a reversed alcohol series: 100%, 96%, 70% and 50% alcohol. A section, thus treated, reveals more of the structures of the tissues, but it still does so in a rather unsatisfactory way. The section must be *stained.*

STAINING

While stains are available for numerous purposes of histologic study, one of the most commonly used stains is hematoxylin and eosin in combination *(H & E).* The components of this stain react chemically with the tissue components. The acid components of the tissue are selectively stained with hematoxylin, whereas the alkaline components are selectively stained with eosin.

Hematoxylin-stained components are purplish blue: all nuclei of cells, some components of cartilage ground substance, granules in the granular layer cells of keratinized, stratified squamous epithelium. Eosin-stained components are pink: protein-rich structures such as the cytoplasm of some cells and collagen fibers, bone matrix.

MOUNTING

Finally, the sections are covered with an extremely thin *cover glass,* but not until the water of the stains, in which the section had been submerged, is replaced, this time with a *mounting medium.* At present, most mounting media are synthetic.

Once again, the sections are run through an alcohol series (70%, 96%, 100%) and xylene. They are then covered with a drop of the mounting medium. A thin cover glass is now gently placed over the medium. The result is a section in mounting medium, sandwiched between two glass slides.

Why is a mounting medium used?

1. To prevent the section from coming into contact with the air. This would cause a fast fading of the histologic stain.

2. To protect the section itself against any physical harm.

3. To make the section truly transparent, which facilitates its study.

HISTOLOGIC TECHNIQUES FOR CALCIFIED TISSUES

An additional step has to be added to this histologic procedure when hard (calcified) tissues, such as dental tissues or bone, are present in the specimen. In that case, *immediately after fixation,* the specimen is *decalcified,* usually in a mildly acid solution. When all the calcium salts have been removed, the acid is washed from the specimen, and the specimen then is treated according to the usual histologic technique, already described.

GROUND SECTIONS (OF UNDECALCIFIED HARD TISSUES)

A second, commonly used, technique to make sections of calcified tissues is the preparation of *ground sections.* The process of decalcification of a hard tissue, as already described, is essential if one wants to make thin paraffin sections. Calcium salts are much harder than paraffin, and their presence in paraffin-embedded specimens may cause substantial disruptions of the sections and damage of the microtome knives.

However, the removal of calcium salts from the calcified tissues may bring about certain changes in the remainder of these tissues, which may be undesirable. In fact, in a highly calcified tissue, such as dental enamel, there is so little ground substance present that it is completely washed away during the process of decalcification. To study enamel with the light microscope, one depends almost exclusively on unstained, undecalcified ground sections (20 to 50 μm thick).

The technique of preparing ground sections is as follows, with the tooth taken as an example:

1. Fixation (formaldehyde solution, 10%).

2. A gross cut is made through the tooth with a fast rotating diamond wheel, under running water.

3. The cut surface of the tooth is polished with progressively finer grades of sandpaper.

4. A second cut is made, parallel to the first one, with the diamond wheel.

5. The resulting thick slab of tooth is now mounted, polished surface down, on a glass slide, with the help of a mounting medium.

6. Now, the unpolished surface of the section is ground on *rough* sandpaper. When the slab is as thin as you want it, and as thin as is physically possible, polishing is completed with progressively finer grades of sandpaper.

7. After thorough washing and drying, a cover glass is mounted over the ground section, in a manner similar to the one used for paraffin sections, using mounting medium. This medium renders the section transparent and allows it to be studied, even though it is considerably thicker than a paraffin section.

INTERPRETATION OF SECTIONED STRUCTURES

In histologic sections, we frequently study structures whose dimensions exceed the thickness of the sections themselves, or are
located near the section plane and have been cut through. In
studying histologic sections, one has to keep this problem in mind

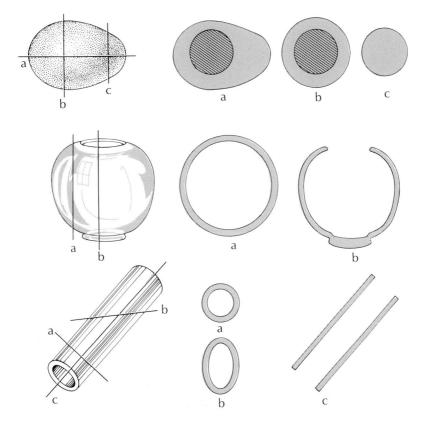

*Fig. A–2. Possible appearance of sections through a hard-boiled egg (top), a bowl
(middle) and a short, cylindrical tube (bottom). The intact structures are shown to the left.
On each, planes of sections (marked with a, b, or c) are indicated. The sections through the
egg are easily tested at home. The sections through the bowl and tube are self-explanatory.
Try to think of possible sections through other structures (an orange, for example). In
histology, it is important to be able to interpret a structure from its sectioned appearance.*

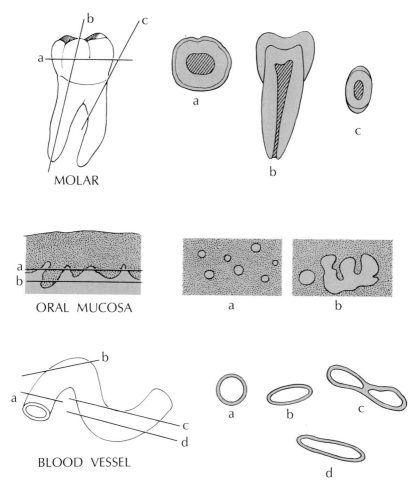

Fig. A–3. *Appearance of sections through a molar tooth (top), a small piece of oral mucosa (middle), and a blood vessel (bottom). Section a through the anatomic crown of a molar consists of a central core of pulp, surrounded by dentin and a thin, peripheral layer of enamel. Section b passes through the entire length of a tooth and one of its roots. Section c consists of a central core of pulp, a layer of dentin and a peripheral layer of cementum. The cementum at the top and bottom of the section is wider than the actual cementum width because of the obliqueness of the section. The horizontal cuts through the oral mucosa both have been made at the level of the interface between epithelium and connective tissue. Section a passes largely through epithelium and only the cross sections through the rounded tops of the connective tissue papillae are included. Section b passes through a large area of connective tissue, while the lower parts of some taller epithelial rete pegs are included in the section as well. Finally, various sections through an irregularly curving blood vessel are shown: a, a true cross section; b, an oblique section, but close to a cross section; d, also an oblique section, but closer to a longitudinal section, and c, a typical section through a curving blood vessel, looping into and out of the section.*

constantly. In Figures A–2 and A–3, it is shown how some structures in a histologic section should be interpreted for their three-dimensional appreciation. We show first how some simple structures would appear in a variety of cuts. Then we show the appearance of structures that could be found in histologic sections, in some of their typical cuts.

SELECTED READING LIST

Möllring, F.K.: *Microscopy from the Very Beginning.* Oberkochen (West Germany), Carl Zeiss, Microscopy Department.
Thompson, S.W.: *Selected Histochemical and Histopathological Methods.* Springfield, Ill., Charles C Thomas, 1966.

INDEX

Page number in *italics* indicate illustrations; those followed by t indicate tables.